INTEF

FASTING

for Women

The Smartest Diet to Lose Weight Fast and Heal Your Body by Eating Healthy. Increase Your Energy, Burn Fat, Optimize Cell Autophagy, Prevent Cancer and Diabetes.

Mely Johnson

Success does not consist in never making mistakes but in never making the same one a second time.

(George Bernard Shaw)

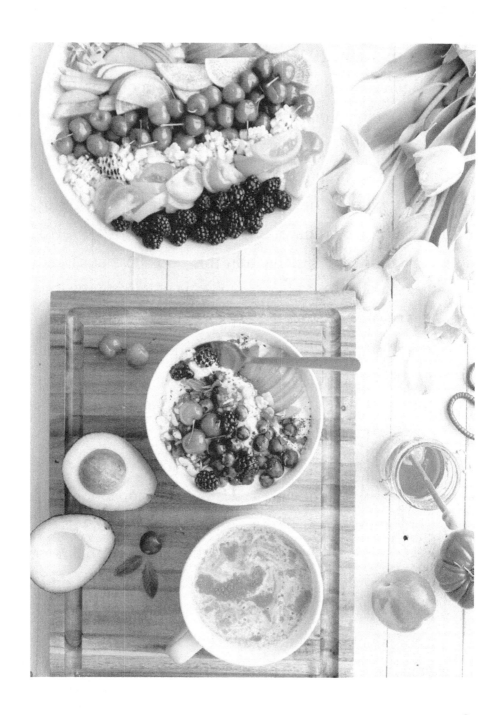

TABLE OF CONTENTS

INTRODUCTION

Intermittent fasting has become one of the world's most common fitness trends. Many people are now using it as a method of losing weight and improving their health. Weight is not gained in a day; hence, you cannot also lose it as quickly. Recent studies have shown that it can have potent effects on the body and brain and even make you live longer. Most people have tried a couple of weight-loss diets in the past that never yielded any results or also if it did, it was a minimal unnoticeable change. The research in this book has been carefully and thoroughly done to give our readers all the information they need to know about intermittent fasting and what they will achieve from the fast. Obesity can bring about diseases such as type 2 diabetes making such patients look for ways to lose a considerable amount in a short period. One of such methods is intermittent fasting. Intermittent fasting is an eating pattern whereby you alternate between eating and fasting. The reason why it is the most preferred weight loss diet is that during the eating period, you are not under strict instruction to eat specific foods. However, during the eating window, always aim for low carb meals to ensure you lose maximum weight during the diet. Contrary to what people may think, intermittent fasting is quite easy, and most people have reported feeling better and having increased energy levels.

CHAPTER 1

WHAT IS INTERMITTENT FASTING?

Intermittent fasting is one of the best health and fitness trends that involve eating and fasting in cycles. It does not stipulate what you should eat, but when to eat and how. It makes intermittent fasting more of an eating pattern rather than a diet. Intermittent fasting helps in the improvement of your metabolism, protection against diseases, reduction of blood sugar levels, and the best one is losing weight. It is also true that intermittent fasting can reduce heart disease. The most common methods of fasting entail 16 or 24hour fasts which can be done two times a week. Throughout evolution, fasting has been practiced by the early man because they were hunters and gatherers, and they couldn't always find anything to eat. It resulted in them functioning for long periods without food. While we sleep, it is said that we are already fasting. Intermittent fasting simply comes in whereby you extend the fast by not having breakfast and eating your first meal of the day at midday and your last meal by 8 pm. It will mean that you are doing the 16hour fast and eating within the 8 hour window period. Intermittent fasting is not as hard as people think, and most people feel more energetic when fasting. In the beginning, it may be difficult to fast since the body is still not used to going for long periods without food, but after a short while, you will find out how easy it is to fast. Religious or spiritual purposes are also another reason for fasting. Usually, during a fast, no food is allowed. Only beverages that have no calories, such as water, coffee, or green tea is allowed. Supplements are also permitted when fasting as long as they don't have calories in them.

Methods of intermittent fasting

There are methods of intermittent fasting whereby you can split the days or weeks into a cycle of eating and fasting. When fasting, you eat minimal amounts of food or nothing at all. Some of the most popular methods of intermittent fasting are 16/8, the 5:2 diet and eat-stop-eat.

i. 5:2 way

The 5:2 fasting method is whereby you consume meals with less than 600 calories on two days of the week, which are not successive.

ii. 16/8 method

The 16/8 method is whereby you eat within 8 hours. It comes about by skipping breakfast and eating from 1 pm to 9 pm and fast for the next 16 hours. The 16/8 method is also known as lean gains protocol.

iii. Eat-stop-eat method

The eat stop eat plan involves not eating for 24 hours. It is whereby one should not eat from, let's say dinner today until the next dinner.

iv. 20:4 method

It is whereby you fast for 20 hours in a day then use the 4 hours to eat a three-course meal.

What effects do intermittent fasting on the body's cells and hormones?

When you go without food for a while, several things happen in your body, especially on the molecular and cellular levels. For instance, stored fat will be made more accessible by the change of hormones levels, which will prompt the body to repair the cells, and in turn, cause gene expression. Below are some of the ways intermittent fasting affects the body's cells and hormones.

i. The rebuilding of the cells.

When fasting, your cells begin the cellular repair process by creating a membrane whereby old and dysfunctional proteins that also build up inside the cells are eliminated. Dead and diseased cells are also not spared. Now the resulting molecules are used to create new healthy cell parts. This whole process is known as autophagy. In layman's language is whereby the body feeds on itself. This process alone plays a role in inflammation control and immunity-boosting. Studies have shown that autophagy protects the body cells against cancer, infections, aging, and above all, insulin resistance. This process makes us more efficient by removing cells that are not adequately functioning and also keeps at bay metabolic dysfunctions such as diabetes and obesity.

ii. Insulin

Insulin resistance is brought about by your body, not being able to identify the hormones that store glucose. Intermittent fasting increases insulin sensitivity, which helps in reducing your chances of getting type2 diabetes as well as burning fat, which is made easily accessible.

iii. Human growth hormone

The human growth hormones help in burning body fat and repairing the muscle mass. They are usually not easily detectable. When you eat from morning to evening, you will not allow many opportunities for the growth hormones to repair your muscles. Fasting stimulates the secretion of human growth hormones. It is usually produced in the pituitary gland and increases the levels of glucose, making it gets suppressed during feeding. The human growth hormones can help in the fast healing of the muscles due to its anabolic effect making the hormone very important for athletes.

iv. Expression of the genes.

Research has shown that intermittent fasting helps against neurodegenerative diseases and expands the life span of a person as well. The beneficial gene changes to protect against infections and give longevity.

v. Intermittent fasting causes an increase in melatonin and decreases the production of cortisol.

Cortisol, which is also known as the stress hormone and the sleep hormone, also known as melatonin, get balanced when doing intermittent fasting. When fasting, people always don't pay attention to the decrease of cortisol and an increase in melatonin. The imbalance of cortisol and melatonin causes weight gain because when you are not well-rested, you get tired the next day which will increase your cortisol level, making you very stressed and fatigued. The good news is, intermittent fasting will quickly help in balancing your hormones.

CHAPTER 2
THE HISTORY OF INTERMITTENT FASTING

Compared to traditional "dieting," fasting is simple and unambiguous. It's always been done. You already unconsciously do IF whenever you skip breakfast or dinner.

Historically, during hunter-gatherer days, our ancestors were in a fasting state while seeking food.

When agriculture was established, civilization came next. But when food was scarce or seasons changed, fasting was still a way of life. Cities and castles stored grain and cured meat for the winter. Before irrigation, lack of rain meant famine, and people fasted to make their stored food last as long as possible until the rains came back, and it was possible for crops to survive again.

Religions flourished in this arrangement of people living closer together, sharing and spreading beliefs and traditions. And religions also prescribed fasting.

Hinduism calls fasting "Vaasa" and observes it during special days or festivals, as a personal penance, or to honor their gods. Islam and Judaism have Ramadan and Yom Kippur when it's forbidden to work, eat, drink, wash, wear leather, and have intercourse. In Catholicism, it's six weeks of fasting before Easter or before Holy Week.

CHAPTER 3

THE SCIENCE OF INTERMITTENT FASTING

To understand the science of Intermittent fasting, we need to look into the basics of nutrition. And it is quite straight-forward: the food we eat gets broken down to molecules and ends up in our blood, which feeds the cells in our bodies. Part of those molecules are net carbohydrates (all carbs in the meal minus the fiber), and our body turns them into sugar (glucose), so our cells could use it for energy.

To be able to use sugar for the energy, we need insulin, which gets produced in our pancreas each time we throw in some food with carbohydrates. Any excess sugars that we don't consume get stored in the form of fat with the idea that we will use that fat for energy later, once we have no sugar left.

The best way how not to end up having substantial fat reserves (and becoming overweight) is to spend the same amount of energy you get from food. However, life is not perfect, and many of us have lifestyles that limit our chances to move throughout the day. Office workers tend to spend 75% of their waking hours sitting.

So, what can we do to lose or not gain weight?

One way to do it is to focus on increasing your energy consumption through increased physical activity or in layman's terms – exercising and doing sports. But you knew this one already, didn't you?

Another way, though, is to focus on consuming less food than you need for the energy that day and as a result, creating a caloric deficit.

And that's where Intermittent Fasting comes in.

Intermittent Fasting makes it easier to reduce the number of meals and calories you eat per day. It's a lot more convenient to not eat at all for some time vs. eating less.

Restricting frequency of meals end up reducing insulin to low enough levels and for long enough time so that our bodies get into the mode of ketosis – a magical state where we use fat for energy vs. sugar. And as a result –

you lose weight. But please be careful – reducing the number of meals or the number of hours you eat per day will only be useful if you consume fewer calories than you need.

The modern era of agriculture and factory-laden "food" (or food-like substances) has completely changed the way humans view and consume food daily, leading to the laundry list of health problems that our society faces today.

Although IF is an ancient practice, the science behind its many health benefits is just recently being exposed to mainstream society. When you fast, you allow your body to cleanse, repair, and regenerate itself for optimal function naturally.

Three of the main health-promoting mechanisms associated with fasting include the metabolic regulation of circadian biology, gut microbiome, and different lifestyle behaviors.

i.Circadian Biology

Humans (and other organisms) have evolved to develop a circadian clock that ensures physiological processes within your body are performed at optimal times throughout the day.

These circadian rhythms occur across 24-hour light-dark cycles and influence changes in biology and behavior.

Interrupting this circadian rhythm negatively impacts metabolism which contributes to obesity and associated diseases such as type 2 diabetes, cardiovascular disease, and cancer.

This is where intermittent fasting comes in.

Feeding signals seem to be the primary timing cue for how your circadian rhythms function and thus control specific metabolic, physiological and behavioral pathways that contribute to overall health, and longevity.

Certain behavioral interventions such as (you guessed it!) intermittent fasting can help synchronize your circadian rhythms leading to improved fluctuations in gene expression, reprogramming of energy metabolism and improved hormonal and body weight regulation, all factors that play a vital role in optimizing your health outcomes.

ii. The Gut Microbiome

The gastrointestinal (GI) tract, better known as the "gut," plays a vital role in regulating several processes within your body.

Many functions of the gut (and nearly every physiological and biochemical function in your body) is influenced by your circadian rhythm described above.

For example, gastric emptying, blood flow and metabolic responses to glucose are greater during the daytime than at night.

So, it's likely that a chronically disturbed circadian rhythm can affect gut function contributing to impaired metabolism and increased risk for chronic disease.

The gut microbiome, also known as our "second brain," has been the subject of extensive research in both health and disease due to its profound involvement in human metabolism, physiology, nutrition, and immune function.

Intermittent fasting has a direct and positive influence on the gut microbiome through:

- Reduced gut permeability
- Diminished systemic inflammation
- Promotion of energy balance by enhancing gut integrity.

Research on both the gut and intermittent fasting continues to emerge while the potential for prevention and treatment of diseases are becoming more widely understood.

iii.Lifestyle Behaviors

Intermittent fasting is shown to help modify different health behaviors such as caloric intake (ie how much you eat), energy expenditure (how much you move), and sleep.

There's no surprise that these three factors contribute to one of the biggest draws to intermittent fasting today: weight loss.

A recent study showed that increasing the nightly fasting duration to greater than 14 hours led to a significant decrease in caloric intake and weight with improvements to:

- Energy levels
- Sleep satisfaction
- Satiety at bedtime

Intermittent fasting also reduces nighttime eating, which contributes to poor sleep quality and reduced sleep duration leading to insulin resistance and increased risk of obesity, diabetes, cardiovascular disease, and cancer.

Fasting puts adaptive cellular stress on the body which in turn allows your body to cope with more severe stressors that may occur and thus protect against potential disease progressions.

This concept is known as hormesis – when exposed to mild stress causes cells in your body to become more resilient against other, more severe stressors.

Think of it this way – what doesn't kill you does make you stronger!

CHAPTER 4
BENEFITS OF INTERMITTENT FASTING

Intermittent fasting has many benefits. Most people fast to lose weight, but for others, it is out of necessity due to lack of food. Sometimes due to illness, human beings, and even animals fast unconsciously. Our bodies can go for long periods without food because it is well fortified and there is nothing strange about that. Intermittent fasting can greatly improve your health as it is a simple way of losing weight and does not require the extensive stress of preparing meal plans. Below are some of the benefits of intermittent fasting.

Intermittent fasting helps in loss of belly fat and weight loss.

Intermittent fasting helps in weight loss by lowering the levels of insulin in the body. Carbohydrates are broken down into glucose, which is used for energy by the cells. The cells can take in glucose thanks to the insulin hormone. When a person is not consuming food, insulin levels drop significantly. Most people doing intermittent fasting are doing it for the sake of losing weight. You will end up taking fewer calories when on the fast. More extended fasting periods make people dig into their stored fats quickly hence making losing the fat easily. The breakdown of body fat is usually facilitated by lower insulin levels and higher growth hormone levels. They ensure the broken down fats are used as energy. It shows that when you fast for a short time, your metabolic rate is increased by 3.6 to 14% when it helps you burn more and more calories. Intermittent fasting is advantageous because as your metabolic rate increases, the amount of food you consume decreases. Studies have now revealed that a person can lose up to 8% in 3-24 weeks. Intermittent fasting works best in losing belly fat, whereby during your eating window, you avoid consuming foods that have too many calories.

Intermittent fasting lowers the risk of diabetes type 2

Diabetes prevention is one of the advantages of going the intermittent fasting way. Due to losing weight while during fasting, other aspects that are related to the risk of suffering from diabetes type 2 reduces. One of the most common ways of suffering from diabetes type 2 is by being overweight. Blood glucose and insulin levels in people who are at risk of diabetes are lowered immensely by intermittent fasting, and the pancreas will not work as it is supposed to. Intermittent fasting has been proved to lower the blood sugar levels, which make the benefits of insulin resistance even more. The reduction of diabetes makers, such as insulin sensitivity, was noted in people who were overweight. A study was carried out on rats that showed that intermittent fasting also protects against kidney damage, which is among the severest problems of diabetes. It only shows that intermittent fasting is a good thing for individuals who are at risk of suffering from diabetes type 2.

Improved heart health

Intermittent fasting has been proved to keep at bay the world's number one killer who is heart disease. Aspects of cardiovascular health is significantly improved by intermittent fasting. Studies show that in both human beings and animals, fasting can help reduce heart rate, cholesterol, and blood pressure. Blood pressure is one of the most prevalent illnesses, and it's a risk factor for other cardiovascular diseases such as kidney disease and stroke. The effectiveness of intermittent fasting in lowering blood pressure was tried in animals first before it was tried on human beings, and it worked perfectly. Another one of the influencing factors of a dysfunctional heart is obesity and other metabolic syndromes. Ketones are usually the primary fuel that gives the body energy. Body mass is generally decreased by the lipids being biochemically transformed, making the total cholesterol concentration to reduce. Intermittent fasting benefits were also looked at when it came to the prevention of hypertension.

Cancer risk reduction

Cancer is usually a disease caused by cells that grow without control. Recent studies show that intermittent fasting could help in delaying how cancer tumors start.

Studies also reasoned that when fasting, the production of blood glucose goes down, and renewal of the immune system when the stem cells are triggered. Cancer growth rate or the possibility of having cancer is also decreased by the intake of healthy and nutritional meals when fasting, and also this enables the production of cells that kill the tumors. One of the significant risks of suffering from cancer is obesity. Fasting helps in the reduction of chances to suffer from obesity, which also leads to type 2 diabetes. The research was extensively carried out in 2016, and the researchers were confident to construe that chemotherapy and fasting together actually slows down the spread of both breast and skin cancer. When the treatment is done together, the levels of the lymphoid progenitor cell production increases. The study also showed that cancer cells are made sensitive to chemotherapy due to starvation, whereas there is the production of the stem cells, and the healthy cells are protected.

Intermittent fasting is good for the brain because it stimulates the creation of new brain cells. Recent studies also have the production of new brain cells means you automatically improve your brainpower. It has been proved that fasting also enhances the rate at which the created brain cells grow and develop the nerve tissue in a process known as neurogenesis. The higher the neurogenesis rate, the better the brain performs. Good brain performances mean that a person is focused; they have a good memory and always in a good mood. The rate of neurogenesis will not only grow during intermittent fasting but also the production of BDNF, which is a crucial protein will be increased. BDNF has been proved to play a significant role in helping the brain to continue to change and adapt. Neuroplasticity usually makes the brain acclimatize to change and be more resilient towards stress. BDNF, which is boosted by intermittent fasting, also supports the neuron functions that are already in existence. Neurological conditions are also avoided as intermittent fasting helps in suppressing brain inflammations. In animals, the fasting was seen to

38

assist in the reduction of neurological disorders like Parkinson's disease, Alzheimer's disease, and even stroke. Intermittent fasting also helps in improving anti-oxidant functions. Mitochondrial replication is also stimulated by starvation, and it has excellent benefits to the brain and its day to day function.

Reduced inflammation

Inflammation is whereby your body protects itself from infections and diseases. Intermittent fasting reduces inflammation significantly. Production of white blood cells, cytokines, and immune cells is increased to help the body fight infections as part of inflammation response. Many chronic illnesses, such as Alzheimer's disease, type 2diabetes, and dementia, are usually caused by excessive inflammation. Swelling, heat, and pain are some of the short-term signs of inflammation. Long term inflammation, on the other hand, always occurs in your body, whereas you will not quickly notice the signs and symptoms, unlike the acute or short-term inflammation. The long-term inflammation, unfortunately, can cause diabetes, cancer, heart disease, and fatty liver disease. Too much stress can also cause long term inflammation. Even overeating sugar can lead to obesity. Recently, scientists found out that eating excessive amounts of refined carbohydrates may lead to inflammation and obesity and insulin resistance. Trans fats have also been proved to cause inflammation, and this is usually brought about by mostly eating processed foods. The trans fats are also known to damage the cells that line up the arteries. Another culprit is the vegetable oil which, when consumed regularly, May result in omega 6 to omega 3 to be imbalanced, which can, therefore, cause inflammation. Another source of inflammation on the body is the intake of excessive red meat and alcohol. Below are some of the methods that intermittent fasting reduces inflammation.

Insulin sensitivity

Studies show that fasting helps to resolve insulin resistance. Inflammation is caused in the body when it resists insulin, and the insulin builds up in the blood. Intermittent fasting usually allows your body to take a break. Due to the lack of food to be digested, insulin levels begin to drop since all the sugar stores in your body are used up.

When fasting, the body uses fat for fuel because it will have used up all the sugar stores. Ketones are created when fats are broken down by the body. Arthritis can be prevented by intermittent fasting because when ketones are produced because the immune systems that regulate the inflammatory disorders are blocked.

Anti-aging

Intermittent fasting causes anti-aging. It slows the rate of aging by setting in motion a chain of events that give the muscles protection. Calorie restriction is the most efficient way of dealing with aging. For more extended periods, traditional calorie restriction and intermittent fasting will cause your body to reduce calories by 20-40%. When you get to your twenties, you will start to experience the growth hormone deficiency. Over time when the growth hormone begins to decline, you will start to feel and even looking older than before. When fasting for 16-24 hours, a high flow of growth hormones will be released. A recent study that was carried out indicated that in women, the growth hormone released was around 1200%, which is 800% less than the human growth hormone produced in men. Always be keen and listen to your body and act accordingly. When the hunger becomes too much, you are allowed to eat but in moderation. With age, comes the decline of hormones. That is where the growth hormones coms in as it protect your organs from aging. Another advantage of the growth hormone is that it improves circulation hence giving a more favorable cholesterol profile. The growth hormone also promotes the repair and recovery of muscles by increasing the synthesis of new protein tissue. The best feature of the growth hormones is that it immensely decreases aging.

The truth about intermittent fasting

Unlike other weight loss programs, intermittent fasting requires very minimal effort, time, and money. All you do is stay away from food. And when the time comes when you are supposed to eat, you eat very minimal quantities in a specific time frame. There are usually ways of going about the diet. To better understand intermittent fasting, you are required first to understand what happens anytime you eat. The hormone insulin is usually released anytime we have our meals. In layman's language, intermittent fasting is unlocking your fat store by letting your insulin levels go down to normal. Unless the insulin levels are down, no weight can be lost. When trying intermittent fasting for the first time, it may be a little bit hard as some may even experience hunger pangs. People are advised to start small by trying different kinds of intermittent fasting to find out what works best to reach their goals. Within the first two weeks of starting intermittent fasting, people will notice things like the grumbling of the stomach. Some people get exhausted and even become shaky due to reduced blood sugar levels when fasting. Some people will become light-headed and feel a void. Most people experience different indications of hunger when fasting. For some, they will not be able to concentrate on anything while others will experience mood swings throughout the day. Other people will be very irritable and even always feel dizzy. People who are fasting and operating heavy machinery or doing heavy work should ensure that they are very alert at all times, and that they are always hydrated and well-rested. Once you have fasted for a month, your body will adjust, and you will feel less hungry and can even go for more extended periods without eating. Some people may complain about the side effects of intermittent fasting. What they need to know is that fasting is just like exercise when you have not done it in a while, you will get out of shape, but your body will soon adjust. Both your body and brain will start feeling better once you get used to fasting. Eating at night is the surest way to gain weight. It is because when you eat at night, the food mostly becomes fat. One of the primary reasons that people start to fast is for weight loss. Most of the people who have made the fasting boast of boosted energy, slimmer body, and a general feel-good feeling. People are encouraged to eat healthy during the eating window and not use intermittent fasting as a justification for eating unhealthy foods during the eating window. Studies have always shown that plant-based diets are usually the best. It does not necessarily mean that you must be vegan; it only means that you should be eating plants more. You can take meat at times or even cake if you like but in moderation. Always make plants take up most of

44

your meals every day. Plants are usually full of proteins, full of fiber, and it will keep you from inflammation. When on these meals, your cholesterol levels will decrease, and it will also immensely improve your digestion. A research that was carried out for a decade showed that eating plant diets can make you live longer as it improves physical health and also emotional health. The best part is that by losing weight, you will not have to worry about cardiovascular health. It will also prevent you from type 2 diabetes and lower your chances of blood pressure. A grand experiment was done on rats to show if intermittent fasting can make animals live longer. It showed that rats that fed less food lived longer. Intermittent fasting usually repairs the pathways hat make animals live longer. Calorie restriction often prevents age-related diseases that include cardiovascular diseases, diabetes type 2, dementia, and even tumors. It means that your life span will increase.

Some of the risks of intermittent fasting

It is always good to listen to your body, especially when it sends out the hunger signals as ignoring this sometimes has consequences. You don't have to be very strict with yourself. You can, at times, choose to eat, though in moderation. People who have suffered from eating disorders can, at times, binge eat. People who have suffered from eating disorders should seek advice from health professionals first before embarking on intermittent fasting. Pregnant women, people on medication, diabetic people, and those who are over 65 are not advised to fast as they continuously need to require food.

Autophagy

Autophagy is the process by which the body cleans out dysfunctional cells to help produce newer cells that are healthier. Auto means 'self' whereas phage means 'eat.' Autophagy means that

When the body doesn't get other sources of food, it begins to devour itself. People usually fast for weight loss and to control their weight, but they use autophagy to help in disease protection. Research has shown that autophagy can be used to protect against diseases such as cancer. Autography happens the most in the very last stages of a long fast. Intermittent fasting has been found to accelerate autophagy to cleanse even more than it would on regular days. Anti-aging is one of the most benefits of autography. Autophagy also helps your metabolism to work at its best by replacing different cell parts. The most important is the mitochondria that act as cell engines that burn fat.

There are usually lots of build ups that are toxic in the mitochondria that can damage cells. By breaking them down using autophagy, you help prevent them from the wear and tear they might get in the future. Healthier cells always work better not only to make proteins but also to burn fuel. Autophagy also works best in ensuring that cell death, which is also known as apoptosis, is minimized. Unlike autophagy, cell death is usually muddled hence the need to clean up. Inflammation is generally triggered by the body to do some cleanup. When renewing tissue, less inflammation will be involved when the cells repair themselves before, they are damaged severely. Another good thing about autophagy is that it improves your skin health. Stuff like air pollution, heat, light, and cold sometimes may damage our skin. The skin can age due to the accumulation of toxins. Autophagy helps one to glow by repairing the existing cells even though the body can make new ones. Autophagy is also functional as it prevents cancer. Chronic inflammation is one of the causes that can make someone have cancer. Autophagy ensures that the process is suppressed. The disease sometimes triggers autophagy when it progresses to hide from the immune system and to get more fuel.

Autophagy also easily supports a healthy weight. It ensures that the toxins in your care reduced. Autophagy also processes energy and packaged proteins hence the metabolic efficiency. It ensures that fats are burned to be used again and spares proteins. Muscle performance is also improved, thanks to autophagy. The muscles are usually inflamed during exercise hence the need for repair. The demand for energy will increase, and this is where autophagy will come in by ensuring the energy required to use the muscle reduces.. Another good thing about autophagy is that it helps in the fight of infectious diseases such as tuberculosis and HIV. When needed, the recruitment of the immune response can be assisted by autophagy. Autophagy can also ensure that microbes are removed from the cells. When proteins around your brain cells don't work right, it makes the aging brain to take more extended periods before they develop. Some proteins do not perform appropriately, so autophagy ensures that they are all cleaned up. For instance, People with Alzheimer's disease have amyloid, which autophagy removes. Autophagy was used in ancient times to preserve life. When you are extremely stressed, the process starts to work hard to repair your cells while minimizing damage. Glucose intruders that are infected can be starved by doing both intermittent fasting and activating autophagy. The fact that autophagy also reduces inflammation means that the immune system will take very minimum time to act in repairing the damage caused by infections. However, as much as autophagy helps in fighting cancer, recent studies have shown that it can have a double effect by making the tumors to resist radiation. It is safe to say that autophagy has dual roles in the fight against cancer. It can act by either suppressing disease or making the tumor grow even more prominent. For cancer patients, weight loss by induced fasting may be harmful. Autophagy is usually induced in all organs when doing intermittent fasting. When people lose weight, they will not need surgery to remove the excess skin since the body will eat it. A study in 2016 carried out on women who had suffered breast cancer, and it showed that there was a low recurrence rate for the once who was able to fast for 14hours in a day. Many people feel like autophagy induced fasting is an eating disorder. The truth is, not necessarily. Today, many people fast for various reasons and some even for health reasons. Some fast so as to help them to retain their muscles. Healthy people are recommended to at least fast for either 36, 48, or 72 hours at least twice a year to induce autophagy. There has not been a way to measure precisely how autophagy is happening in a body as this will not give the exact readings. It is because of the rise and fall of some tiny protein ratios. A study in 2017 showed that it is not possible to measure autophagy in humans.

CHAPTER 5
TECHNIQUES OF INTERMITTENT FASTING

In recent years, intermittent fasting has gained so much popularity in the fight against obesity. Intermittent fasting involves avoiding food or eating during a stipulated time before going back to regular consumption. Recent studies show that this type of eating pattern has various advantages, such as increased longevity, weight loss, and good health. When embarking on the intermittent fasting journey, preparation is essential. To maintain a healthy weight and an excellent metabolic profile should be the most crucial goal of intermittent fasting. Discipline is vital so as not to get tempted to indulge in free feeding. It is not as easy to fast, especially when you go to events and they have prepared delicious meals. For you to be a bit wary of the food you eat and the number of calories they have, you can download applications on your phone that counting calorie before you indulge in meals. Also, when preparing meals, ensure that plant diets are more on your plate.

Above all, your attitude towards intermittent fasting is what will limit your success. As hard as it may seem, it is undoubtedly possible. Every person's experience with intermittent fasting is different due to the various individual lifestyles. Below we will talk about the different intermittent fasting techniques and how to make it a lifestyle.

12-hour fasting

It is whereby an individual needs to decide on when to fast within 12 hours. Researchers found that the body will burn its stored fats into energy when you go on a 10-16 hour fast. This process will help in the release of ketones into the bloodstream, which will then cause a person to lose weight. For beginners, this will be the best option of fasting since the fasting window is quite small. Much fasting usually occurs when someone is asleep, and each day, the person is allowed to consume the same number of calories. So, for example, if you ate dinner at 9 pm, you are allowed to have breakfast at 9 am the following day. You to go through the 12hour fast period smoothly, make sure you include your fasting window in your sleep.

The 12-hour fasting techniques have many health benefits. Some of them are;

i.   Detoxification.

The body is known to use lots of energy to ensure that it removes toxins from your body. The body usually focuses on eliminating toxins and healing itself when it is not digesting food, and that's why the 12 hour fast is essential. Detoxification is optimized because when you go on the loose, the body will focus on repairing itself.

ii.   Helps in managing weight.

For the body to burn its glycogen supply, it will take roughly 8 hours. When the number of glycogen finishes, the body will use the stored fats to produce energy. It becomes a bit hard for the body to burn fat when someone eats throughout the whole day. When you stay for 12 hours without eating, the body taps in the fat reserve forcefully to produce energy.

iii. Research shows that fasting can significantly improve the health of the mitochondria.

Brain health immensely enhances through the support of mitochondrial health. Recent studies have also demonstrated that progressive brain disorders might be prevented thanks to intermittent fasting.

The 16/8 method

During the 16/8 way, you are supposed to fast for 16 hours and only eat during an 8-hour window. For someone who has already tried the 12hour fast, this method will not be hard. In this technique, men usually fast for a good 16 hours, while women are allowed to go for 14 hours. It is because research shows that women do better with shorter fasts. Within the eating window, you can feed on two to three meals. The 16/8 technique can also be called a lean gains protocol. You can have the last meal for supper the fast until lunchtime the following day. It might be a bit hard to get used to in the beginning, especially for people who like having breakfast, but as you continue, it becomes easier. To reduce hunger levels, you are allowed to have water, coffee, and other beverages that do not contain calories. Ensure that you do not use sugar, cream, or milk as they are known to provide calories. If you eat loads of junk that have thousands of calories during your eating window, you will not see results. You are supposed to eat healthy meals. A balanced diet consists of veggies, fresh fruits dairy nuts, and beans. You can also have lean meat. Even eating meals that are low in carbs may help blunt your appetite. When you are on the 16/8 fast, make sure you stay hydrated as this will significantly reduce hunger levels. For you to burn body fat while holding on to muscle, you have to keep active.

24 hours fast weekly.

The 24 hours weekly fast is also known as the eat-stop-eat diet. It is whereby you fast from one dinner and eat during the next dinner. However, it can also be done by fasting from breakfast to breakfast or from lunch to lunch. During the fast, you are only allowed water, coffee, or any beverage that does not have calories. If you are doing the 24hour fast for weight loss, then ensure during the eating period, you consume food generally as if you have not been fasting. You, however, do not have to start with the 24hour fast; you can begin with 14 or even 16hours. Most people always complain of hunger during the last hours of the fast. For you to finish a 24hour diet plan, you have to be much disciplined.

5:2 fasting technique.

The 5:2 fasting technique is whereby you eat for five days in a week, as usual, then the remaining two days you feed on meals that have below 500 calories. Most people like separating their fast days throughout the week. For example, you can fast on Saturday and Wednesday and regularly eat during the other days of the week. For more exceptional results, ensure there is a day you do not fast between your fasting days. The research which has been done on obese women agreed that when you restrict calories twice a week, it leads to weight loss. The participants also had reduced insulin levels, which significantly impacted their insulin sensitivity. There is no rule on what to eat on fasting days or when to eat it. The time people prefer to eat vary as some may wish to eat a small meal at breakfast while others may prefer eating as later during the day. People always follow two meal plans, which are, three meals spread across the day, and two meals spread across the day. You are advised to use your calories well since you have a minimal intake of calories. When having your meals, try and consume foods that are high in fiber and proteins as they will help you to feel full without eating many calories. During fast days, it is said that when you consume soups, you will be fuller than the original ingredients. For fast days, you can have;

- Vegetable or tomato soup
- Sparkling water
- Natural yogurt
- Black coffee
- Black tea
- Large portions of veggies.

It is usually good to experiment what works best for you as there is no specified for eating when fasting. It is usual to feel extremely hungry during fast days. When you keep busy or run errands, the hunger pangs slowly fade, and sometimes you even feel like you have eaten. When you fast for a couple of times, it gets better and better every time you do it. Someone who is just starting is often advised to have a simple snack just in case the hunger becomes too much, and you begin to feel ill. Not everyone can do intermittent fasting. Only well-nourished and healthy people are allowed to fast. Some of the people who should avoid intermittent fasting are;

- Malnourished people who have a history of nutrients deficiency.

- Pregnant and nursing mums.

- People who are suffering from type 1 diabetes

- Women who have fertility issues

- People who have eating disorders.

Alternate day fasting. (ADF)

It is one of the techniques used to do intermittent fasting. On this technique, you are allowed to fast every other day, but on the days, you are not fasting, you can eat whatever you want. Some people usually avoid food totally during the fast days, or they take meals which have not more than 500 calories. Some people may also choose to feed as much as they want on feeding days. For beginners, this may be a bit hard since you need to fast for long hours. What you are required to do is fast on one day and eat as much as you want on the following day. During the days of the fast, you can drink beverages that do not have calories such as coffee, black tea, and water. The studies about alternate fasting that were carried out showed that many people preferred alternate fasting to other techniques siting that it was easier. Research that was carried out showed that obese people who practice the alternate day fasting technique, lose up to 7% of their body weight. Alternate day fasting was found to help in the loss of more fat while preserving greater muscle mass. Alternate day fasting and exercise combined help in losing weight faster and twice as much as fasting alone. During fasting days, sometimes a person may get so hungry while at other times, the hunger might not be there. Always be careful about compensatory hunger, which most often makes people overindulge in food during their eating window. It has been proven that compensatory appetite is increased dramatically by continuously restricting calories whereby when on the alternate day fast, it does not increase. Some people who have tried the modified alternate-day method say that when their hunger decreases significantly after two weeks, making the fasting days very easy for them. Alternate day fasting also has been proven to have very positive effects on the body when you are both losing weights and even when maintaining the pressure. One of the most effective ways of preserving muscle mass is by doing the alternate day fast.

Health benefits of the alternate day fasting

Weight loss aside, alternate day fasting has many benefits. Some of the health benefits include;

- Cardiovascular health

When obese people lose weight, it reduces their heart risk factors by minimizing the chances of heart disease. Some of the few universal benefits of alternate-day fasting are that the cholesterol concentration will reduce a great deal. Blood pressure and triglycerides will also reduce significantly.

- ## Diabetes type 2.
In the US, 95% of diabetes always type 2 diabetes. When levels of the blood sugar are high but not high enough to make it be considered diabetes, it is called pre-diabetes. Losing weight acts as one of the ways that restrict diabetes. When it comes to lowering insulin levels and reducing its resistance, alternate day fasting is the best since it has a minimal effect on the control of blood sugars. It has been said that when a person has high levels of insulin, it may cause them to be obese and have cancer.

- ## Autophagy in alternate-day fasting.
When stimulation of autophagy occurs, it is said to be one of the most common effects of the body. It is the process whereby old cells that are not functioning are broken down and recycled. Studies show that autophagy reduces the risk of getting tumors. Alternate days fasting have also been proven to promote longevity and a healthy body.

- Adaptive thermogenesis, which is the effect of a drop in resting metabolic rate, is usually caused by fasting. During the period of fasting whereby you restrict calories, your body will reduce the number of calories it will burn by conserving energy. Therefore, it will make you not to lose weight as expected. The good thing about alternate day fasting, the metabolic rate will not drop. With the alternate fasting, people generally lose weight because you get provided with fewer calories than the body needs.

The 20:4 fasting techniques.

The 20; 4 intermittent fasting method, also known as the worrier diet, is whereby you fast for 20 hours and have your meals within the 4 hours. During the fast, you are not allowed to consume any snacks or beverages that have calories. Sleep usually counts as part of the fast. This diet, unlike other programs that do not allow the intake of carbohydrates, often stresses the idea of timing what you consume and when to drink it. When you fast for long hours like, for example, in the worrier's diet, which is 20 hours, insulin will automatically stay low for a more extended period. All you can have during this time is coffee, tea, or any other beverage that does not have calories. It is not a must for you to limit the eating window to evenings only like it was done before; you can tailor-make your fasting and eating window according to your preferences. When you do the 20:4 fasting techniques, you are sure to be more focused and have more energy. The first days of the fast, you may experience hunger pangs, but when you go on with the fasting, the hunger will tremendously reduce. This technique of intermittent fasting can quickly become addictive once you see the mental clarity that comes with it. Above all intermittent fasting techniques, the worrier's diet seems to be the strictest because it only has a 4-hour eating window, and most people are unable to adhere to that. As we said earlier, you can tailor-make the fast to suit you. Some people who are fasting, prefer to drink morning coffee and leave the 4 hour eating period for evenings. However, some find themselves hungrier during the day hence scheduling their eating window at lunch hour. What you are advised is that it does not matter what time you choose your eating period to be, what matters is that you stick to an extremely low carb diet. Low carbohydrates usually make the hunger pangs to go down, and this will help you get through the 20 hours of fasting. For the 20 hours fast, it is usually advised to stick to the ketogenic diet by eating meals such as;

- For the starches: sweet potatoes, corn, and potatoes.
- For proteins; lean meat, fish, chicken, and eggs are allowed.
- Oats, bread, pasta
- For oils, you can use olive oil
- Milk, cheese, and yogurt.
- Cauliflower, zucchini, leafy veggies.

Always choose foods that are higher in protein to consume fewer fats. Some people have a heavy meal at the beginning of the eating window, and when the eating window is almost, they have a simple snack. Ensure that you have your meals early enough in that when you have your heavy meal, you don't get so full that you feel uncomfortable when going to bed. Glycogen, a carbohydrate in storage form, will be used up when the body has not had anything and especially during your feeding period when you only had ketogenic foods.

Throughout the fasting period, the body will begin to burn more body fat when the glycogen finishes. The longer you stay without eating, the better because your insulin levels will remain low, and this will ensure that the liver uses your body fat to fuel itself. When your blood glucose is low, the liver will be signaled by the little insulin prompting it to dump its glycogen into the bloodstream. The 20:4 fasting techniques have many side effects and benefits. One of the advantages is that you will have reduced cholesterol and inflammation. We have seen all the benefits of inflammation on the other chapters above. When on the 20:4 diet, you will improve mental clarity, and your concentration will be top-notch. Your blood glucose levels will also increase tremendously. If you were used to eating lots of carbohydrates, you will see significant changes as you will not be feeling hungry and craving unhealthy meals. Cases of insulin resistance can be corrected using the 20:4 fasting technique. Fat stores are made more accessible to the liver by reducing your food intake hence lowering your insulin levels.

The 23:1 fasting technique

This technique is also known as OMAD, which stands for one meal per day. People can lose weight by having one meal per day, which is intermittent fasting. It means that you will fast for 23 hours then have a 1 hour period where you can have your lunch. During the fast, you are only allowed to take beverages with zero calories such as coffee, black tea, or green tea, whereas, during your eating period, you can have your regular meals. It is, however, advisable to feed on meals that are rich in nutrients. Apart from weight loss, the 23:1 fasting technique has a lot of health benefits. Some of the health benefits are;

- Decreased rates of contracting diseases
- The human growth hormone increases
- The inflammations levels are lowered drastically
- Autophagy
- Has a positive impact on sleeping patterns of people who are obese
- It helps people with diabetes type 2 to lower their blood sugar levels.

This diet is not as hard to follow because the number of calories is not counted. The effects of the 23; 1 cycle may be a bit different in men because unlike women, they do not go through hormonal cycles. Enhancement of ketosis is also one of the benefits of the 23: 1-hour fasting technique. OMAD is usually a prolonged fast, and thus, it often maximizes n benefits such as anti-inflammatory, fat-burning, and autophagy. Due to the long hours without food, the 23:1 fasting technique might have some downside. Some of the disadvantages are:

- **Not getting enough food.**

The OMAD diet or 23:1 diet means that you fast for long hours, which makes it hard at times for the body to get enough food. For you to ensure that you are well sorted during the fasting window, always ensure that you eat food that has calories. Ensure that the calories you eat are enough for your weight, age, and the type of activities you carry out daily. Also, ensure that the meal you eat during your feeding period is one heavy meal. When you are not used to intermittent fasting, the 23:1, not getting enough food may cause you to lose focus.

- **Another downside of OMAD is that it can cause extreme hunger.**

Due to the long periods without food, a person may get so hungry when fasting, and this might lead to temptations of feeding on unhealthy foods when you are only supposed to feed on foods that don't have calories.

- **Feeling weak.**

Due to the more extended fasting periods and having just a meal in a day may cause a person to feel weak. It is because the food intake will have decreased, and hence making the body to produce energy that is not enough eventually will lead to fatigue.

- **Getting fewer nutrients.**

Studies have proved that on a day to day basis, a female adult needs 2500 calories, whereas a man needs 2000 calories. When you are on the OMAD or the 23; 1 technique of fasting, you only get only 750 calories hence making a person hungry. To get nutrients such as calcium that usually are not found in the meals, a person is advised to drink yogurt or milk.

-   It causes a person to be irritable.

A person may become easily irritated because of hunger. It is also easy for the person to not concentrate and even have mood swings.

For those who are just starting the intermittent fasting, the OMAD or 23:1 fasting technique is not advisable. You can begin by doing the most straightforward routines, like lowering your sugar intake. Also, try and put your focus on healthy fats and take lots of veggies and clean proteins which will act as a stepping stone towards OMAD fasting.

- **Food you are allowed to eat during intermittent fasting.**

A popular misconception is that you can allow yourself to eat anything while doing Intermittent Fasting, including fast food, sugary, and highly processed dishes. If your goal is to lose weight, improve productivity, and simply get healthier, it is essential to stick to healthy meals.

This means eating whole foods and avoiding the usual suspects such as sugar, processed foods, empty carbs, etc.

The type of diet you choose is up to you; as long it is balanced and fits your lifestyle. For many, the Keto Diet has proven to be a great supplement to Intermittent Fasting, as it may help you burn more fat.

When doing intermittent fasting, there are restrictions whatsoever on the type of foods you should eat when on your feeding window. For the intermittent fasting to be more productive, feed on unprocessed foods that are high in fiber. The menus below are some of the recommended foods that you should take during fasting.

70

i. Avocado.

Unlike other fruits that are high in carbohydrates, avocados contain healthy fats. Just like olive oil, avocados contain monounsaturated fats that always leave a person full for more extended periods after consumption. As much as the avocado fruit high percentage fat, it contains lots of water and fiber. The good thing about avocados is that you can add them to salads. Apart from that, they also contain nutrients that are important to the body and potassium.

ii. Fish.

Fish that have a few fats like the salmon fish are significant during intermittent fasting. It is because, when you eat it, you will remain full for long hours. Apart from quality protein and healthy fats, salmon also contains reasonable amounts of vitamin D. iodine may also be found in fish. The nutrients found in fish are essential because they ensure the thyroid functions properly. When the thyroid functions correctly, it keeps your metabolism running at optimum. When you consume fish, you get the omega3 fatty acids that studies have shown help to reduce inflammations.

iii. Eggs.

In some people, the levels of bad cholesterol increase by consuming eggs. When you are on a weight-loss mission, they are one of the best foods you can eat. It is because it has proteins and you can cook it up in minutes, and it will make you feel full for long hours. For muscle build-up, you need as much protein as possible. You can now get all the nutrients you need on a calorie-restricted diet as eggs are always nutrients dense. Eggs also promote weight loss by suppressing appetite during the day.

iv. Leafy greens

Kales, collards, and spinach, are some of the leafy greens that you should consume during intermittent fasting. They are usually very loaded with fiber and low in carbohydrates, making them extremely good for weight loss. You can comfortable eat a lot of leafy greens without the fear of consuming a lot of calories. The leafy greens also contain minerals and antioxidants. They are also very nutritious and have vitamins. When you take the leafy greens, you will always feel full for longer hours due to the high fiber content.

v. Whole grains.

Some whole grains are very healthy, and this is because they have loads of fiber. It will help in making you feel full for long hours at a time. Some of the examples of whole grains are oats. Oats usually have fiber that is soluble and ensures you stay fuller for longer, and your metabolic health is guaranteed. Resistant starch can be found in white and brown rice, especially when you let it cool down after cooking. Keep off from refined grains as they are not a healthy choice. It also makes them have high carbohydrate levels. Unlike refined grains, whole grain can quickly turn up your metabolism.

vi. Chia seeds.

It is one of the most nutritious foods on earth. The level of fiber in chia seeds is pretty high hence making it one of the foods that have the lowest levels of carbohydrates on the surface. Chia seeds can quickly expand your stomach because of their ability to absorb up to 11 times their water weight due to the high fiber content. According to recent studies done, it was found out that chia seeds that reduce a person's appetite. Due to the type of nutrient composition in chia seeds, it makes them help in weight loss. When you consume chia seeds, you will be full for more extended hours hence.

vii. Legumes

Legumes and beans are usually low-calorie diets. Grains such as chickpeas, black beans, and kidney beans have been proven to assist in weight loss. They have very high fiber and protein content, and these are the two nutrients that enable a person to feel full for longer hours after feeding. It is essential to prepare the legumes well because some people are unable to stand them, and this is because they have resistant starch.

viii. Potatoes.

For optimal health, potatoes seem to have specific properties that ensure that the body is functioning well. They usually contain a very diverse range of nutrients, nearly everything needed by the body. Potassium, which is found in potatoes, has been found to play a significant role in the reduction of blood pressure. When boiled potatoes were put on a satiety index scale that measures how filling foods are, they scored the highest among all the processed foods. What this shows is that when you eat white potatoes, you will feel fuller and have fewer cravings for other foods. A fiber-like substance that is starch resistant will be formed when you boil your vegetables and leave them to cool down. Apart from only weight loss, the fiber-like content can also lead to loss of weight.

ix. Cruciferous veggies.

When you hear about cruciferous veggies, all they mean are vegetables like broccoli, cabbage, and cauliflower. These vegetables are very high in fiber and can make you full for long hours. The other good thing about the cruciferous veggies is that they contain the right amount of protein. They do not provide high protein levels like the ones in animals or even beans, but in the vegetable kingdom, they have the highest protein levels. For weight loss, cruciferous veggies are perfect for you since they have a great combination of low energy density, proteins, and fiber. The other advantage of cruciferous vegetables is that it has substances that were found to be useful in the fight against cancer. Including them in your diet will always improve your overall health.

x. Soups.

For you to eat fewer calories, ensure you consume a meal that has a low energy density. Vegetables and fruits are known to have low energy densities because they contain lots of water. Studies show that when you eat the same food as a soup rather than when it's whole, you feel fuller for longer hours at a time. It will make them eat fewer calories. When added to your soup, the cream can make you consume a lot of calories, so try and avoid it while cooking. For a weight loss diet, soup can be very filling and effective because of the water content.

xi. Tuna.

The tuna is which a low-fat fish is, one of the best high protein foods that have low calories. It is a meal that has high protein levels and low calories and fat level; hence, why it is preferred so much by bodybuilders. Tuna that is put in a can that contains water is better than the one canned in oil since it has higher protein levels. Tuna is lean and has a very high-quality protein.

xii. Apple cider vinegar.

Some people use apple cider vinegar in their drinking water. Among the health community, apple cider vinegar is essential because it can be used for weight loss. When you are having a high carbohydrate meal and apple cider vinegar at the same time can make someone get fuller and eat up to 260 calories less during the day. A research was carried out on obese people, and it was found out that drinking apple cider vinegar made them lose weight. Taking vinegar after meals is also beneficial since it reduces the spike of blood sugar. Another good thing about apple cider vinegar is that it curbs your appetite, especially when you add it to salads. It will, therefore, your weight loss journey effortless.

xiii. Chili pepper.

Chili pepper contains capsaicin a substance that has been proved to reduce appetite tremendously. Some studies also show that it burns fat fast. Many supplements for weight loss use the capsaicin as an ingredient. Eating a gram of chili pepper reduced appetite and increased the fat burning process. Unfortunately for people who are used to eating chili, there was no effect because over time after eating chili, it builds up some tolerance in the body. The heat can increase oxidation of the fat layers in the body in chili pepper.

xiv. Nuts.

Nuts are usually healthy as they contain many nutrients and antioxidants. One of its advantages is that it protects the heart against diseases. They contain calories and fats that help the body with energy. The unsaturated fats found in nuts can also protect the body against many diseases, including heart disease. Most people do not add nuts to their diet because they contain fats hence the fear of weight gain. Recent studies have concluded that eating nuts may not lead to weight gain but lead to weight loss. The study showed that those who ate nuts weekly were better placed to lose weight than those who never ate nuts at all. Whether people follow a rigorous diet or not, eating nuts does not make them add weight. Another reason why nuts are one of the recommended foods during weight loss is that it reduces hunger and makes a person feel fuller for longer. Cravings can also be reduced immensely by snacking on nuts and especially almonds. Hormones like peptide and cholecystokinin are usually produced when someone snacks on nuts. The hormones are known to suppress and regulate appetite. This is because nuts often have high unsaturated fat and protein content. When you snack on nuts and add a few calories, they go through an elimination process that occurs when you eat other foods. Another reason to support the fact that nuts do not add weight is that most of the chewed nuts will undigested and empties as feces making the fats not to be absorbed.

xv. Lean meat.

Despite the lack of evidence, beef has been said that it causes many illnesses. Meat is very high in protein. Unprocessed red meat is very healthy and does not cause any heart diseases — however, unprocessed beef, which is unhealthy for consumption. One of the most filling nutrients is proteins. In a day, you can burn lots of calories just by eating diets that have a high protein level. Unprocessed lean meat can significantly improve your protein levels. For you to lose a substantial amount of weight, you are advised to take a high protein diet instead of carbohydrates.

xvi. Cheese.

When on the weight loss journey, meals high in proteins are essential. Cheese has high protein content and very few fats and carbohydrates. Dairy products also contain calcium, which is one nutrient that helps in weight loss.

xvii. Grapes

Studies have shown that grapefruit contains insulin resistance. Before you eat your daily meals, ensure you start by eating the grapefruit to feel fuller for longer hours. When you eat it before meals, it suppresses your appetite hence reducing the number of calories consumed.

xviii. Yogurt

Most yogurts contain what we call probiotic bacteria. One of its advantages is to improve the gut functions, which in turn protects against inflammation. If the gut functions are not developed, one can suffer from leptin resistance, which is one of the causes of obesity. Recent studies also showed that probiotic yogurts could improve digestive health, making an individual have a reduced risk of obesity.

xix. Coconut oil

Coconut fats are what we call the good fats. It has high levels of fatty acids that when consumed, make someone feel full for more extended periods. Research carried out showed that coconut oil reduced belly fat in both men and women. It is advisable to use coconut oil in cooking rather than the usual cooking fats. Medium-chain triglycerides are usually found in coconut oil, and they are the ones responsible for making a person feel fuller for longer. Another one of the best fats in the world is the extra virgin oil. It is one of the healthiest fats due to cold pressing when produced. The other good thing about the extra virgin oil is that it is unrefined and has many vitamins and minerals. The oils are also good for your heart since they contain monounsaturated fatty acids. The fatty acids also help in the stabilization of blood sugar levels.

- **Foods that you to avoid during intermittent fasting.**

As much as there are no restrictions on how to eat when doing intermittent fasting, it is always advisable to eat healthy meals. Most times, people get confused about healthy and unhealthy snacks. For you to lose weight, you have to avoid certain foods and as it will help in keeping illnesses at bay. Below we shall see all the foods to avoid to stay healthy during and after the fasting period.

i. Fried foods.

Fried foods usually contain calories at high levels. Most restaurants prefer deep frying because it cuts down on costs. As much as many people love fried food, Fried foods are many people's favorite, but these foods are unhealthy because they contain fat. These fats are formed through a process called hydrogenation. What people who manufacture food do, is they use the hydrogenation process to help the processed food last longer. During frying of foods, changes occur on their chemical structure, making it very hard for the body to break it down. Many diseases, such as heart disease, obesity, and diabetes, are usually caused by trans-fats.

Most of the time, vegetable oil is used during deep-frying, which is said to be containing trans-fat even before its heated. Most people reuse frying oil, which makes the level of fats to go up even higher. Eating fried foods often causes the rate of chronic illnesses to go up. Diseases such as obesity and high blood pressure are all illnesses that are mostly caused by fried foods. Studies that were carried out showed that women who ate more than one fish serving per week were at an extremely high risk of heart failure than women who never ate fish often. People who are at a higher risk of suffering from diabetes type 2 are the ones who take fried foods usually. Studies carried out showed that people who are at more risk to suffer from insulin resistance were the ones who consumed fried foods more than two times weekly. It is advisable to consume non-fried foods since they contain fewer calories. The hormones that are used in appetite regulation can be affected by fried foods since they lead to weight gain. Weight gain has not been associated with polyunsaturated and monounsaturated fats. Another disadvantage of frying food is that, during the use of high temperatures to cook, a toxic substance known as acrylamide will be formed. Foods that are rich in fat like potatoes and baked foods are known to contain very high levels of acrylamide. It has also been found that the high levels of acrylamide put one at risk of getting cancer of different parts of the body. People who enjoy fried foods should endeavor to prepare them at the comfort of their homes using healthy oils. Some of the healthy oils include;

- Avocado oil

- Coconut oil

- Olive oil.

Some of the health risks brought about by feeding on fried food can be minimized by using the above oils in preparing your meals. We also have oils that contain high levels of polyunsaturated fats which, when exposed to heat, will form acrylamide. Such oils should avoid at all costs when deep-frying our foods. Examples of such oils are:

- Sunflower oil

- Grapeseed oils

- Sesame oils

- Corn oil

- Canola oil

- Soybean oil.

These oils contain Trans-fats even before heating it and frying your food. The bottom line is that foods cooked in unhealthy oils greatly put your health at risk. Therefore, it is better to avoid eating foods cooked in such.

ii. Beverages containing sugar.

Drinks that contain sugar are typically very harmful because you always take so much as your brain will not record them as food. When we talk about beverages containing sugar, we mean sweetened coffee, sodas, milkshakes et cetera. The reason why sugary drinks are discouraged during intermittent fasting is that it leads to rapid weight gain. When you consume large amounts of sugar, it will be turned into fat by your liver hence gaining weight. When you use large amounts of table sugar, fructose will be supplied to your body. Unlike glucose, which can be broken down by all cells in the body; it will be turned into fat. Fructose does not help you to feel full, and this may lead you to take up lots of calories. People who drink sweetened beverages are always at risk of being obese. Sugar or sweeteners are discouraged because they bring about belly fat. Belly fat, which is also known as visceral fat, can cause diabetes type 2. Sodas may cause your cells to resist insulin effects. Type 2 diabetes and heart disease happen when the body becomes insulin resistant. A lot of studies that have been carried out show that when you consume lots of soda, you can easily suffer from type 2. Sugary beverages do not contain any helpful nutrients. Fat cells in our bodies produce a hormone known as leptin, which is used to control the number of calorie intake and the amount the body burns. Fat gain in humans is caused by leptin resistance. This hormone usually changes with the body when it's either obese or starving.

Another reason we are advised to keep off sugary beverages is that it is addictive. Sugar and hard drugs both affect your brain the same way because they give feelings of pleasure. Taking sugar may cause food addiction. Sugary beverages are also discouraged as they may lead to cardiovascular-related illnesses. It is not a secret that drinks sweetened with sugar can make a person have higher risks of suffering from diseases such as high blood sugar levels. It has also been established that people who drink lots of soda have higher risks of suffering from cancer because of other chronic illnesses such as obesity and diabetes type 2. Comprehensive research was carried out, and it showed that pancreatic cancer was likely to attack people who drank sugary sodas weekly. Sugary sodas are also discouraged because just as bad as they are for weight loss and general health, they are bad for the teeth. Carbonic and phosphoric acids that are found in sodas are nasty for dental hygiene because they make your teeth to decay very quickly. On their own, the acids in sugars are very harmful, and when they combine with sugar, it gets worse. Gout is also one of the health conditions that a person who drinks soda may go through. The carbohydrate fructose is responsible for high uric acid levels in the body. Eventually, the uric acid becomes candied, and that is when a person will start suffering from gout. When the brain is not able to function appropriately, especially in adults, they suffer from diseases such the Alzheimer's disease. When the blood sugar levels are incredibly high, the risk of dementia also rises.

iii. Breakfast cereals.

These are grains that have gone through processing and contain high levels of added sugar. They are usually eaten with milk and are more common in children. Some of the cereals are oats, rice, and even corn. Shredding and roasting ae some of the processes used to ensure the breakfast cereals to be a bit more edible. Most breakfast cereals have very high sugar content. It is advisable to consume grains that have high fiber content and very minimal sugar levels.

iv. Agave nectar

People nowadays have become health conscious, making sweeteners to gain popularity. Agave, which is usually said to be a natural diabetic-friendly sweetener, is one of them. Tequila is also made from agave by fermentation. Agave is not healthy for consumption because of all the processing it goes through. The reason why sweeteners high in fructose are generally said to be healthy is that fructose takes time before it raises the levels of insulin in the body. When you compare agave to regular sugar, you find that all its sugar content is in fructose form hence the very little glucose in it. Agave is not advisable due to its large amounts of fructose. Glucose and fructose serve very different purposes may look similar, but they serve extremely various objects on the body. Healthy foods such as fruits and veggies contain glucose, and just so you have enough, the body ensures it produces glucose. The good thing about glucose is that every living cell in your body can absorb it, unlike fructose, which can only be incorporated in the liver. When you consume large amounts of fructose, your liver gets burdened, and this will cause it to change the fructose into fat. It will, in turn, make the blood triglycerides to rise higher. A research carried out showed that the fats produced can cause something called fatty liver disease due to the fats wedged around it. Fructose was also found to be responsible for insulin resistance, and this occurs, especially when it has been consumed in large quantities for an extended period. Belly fat is another disadvantage of consuming foods high in fructose because it will cause your levels of bad cholesterol will go up.

v. White bread

Bread has been consumed for centuries. It is made from water and flour and yeast. It is considered to be fattening, and unlike fruits and veggies, it has almost zero nutrients. Bread usually comprises of a lot of calories and carbohydrates. Eating it may not add any nutritional value to your body since it has very levels of vitamins and proteins. Most wheat products have gluten, which is usually used to help the dough to rise before baking. Gluten is known to cause harm to the small intestines lining due to an autoimmune disorder. Nutrients absorption in the body is also impaired due to the celiac disease. Gluten sensitivity is also an issue that some people face, and this usually makes them get bloated or even have diarrhea. People with such problems should not consume white bread as this will help them avoid the adverse effects of gluten. Another reason why food is discouraged during fasting is that it has high carbohydrate levels. When you take white bread, blood sugar levels will go up because of the carbohydrate the body breaks down to glucose. When you consume foods that have a high carbohydrate level, it increases your chance to suffer from diseases like diabetes type 2 and other illnesses that might cause the instability of the heart function. Whole grain bread always has high fiber content, which will reduce the speed at which sugar will be absorbed into the bloodstream. It will then ensure that the blood sugar level stabilizes. During the intermittent fasting period, it is advised to stay away from bread because they have anti-nutrients that block anti-nutrients from being absorbed by the body. Phytic acid, which is a molecule that folds itself to essential minerals like zinc and calcium prevents the absorption of these crucial minerals in the body. The gluten and anti-nutrients found in bread may cause very many health issues for most people in the long run.

i. Processed meat

Unlike its unprocessed counterpart, processed meat is very unhealthy. Studies have shown that most illnesses are caused by consuming processed meat. Heart disease, type 2 diabetes, and even colon cancer are some of the conditions that can be caused by processed meat. Processed meats have usually been conserved by canning, smoking, and even curing. Some of the processed meat includes:

- Ham
- Bacon
- Salted meat
- Canned meat
- Sausages
- Salami
- Hotdogs

People who feed on processed meat have been said to take meager amounts of healthy foods such as veggies and fruits. Many long-lasting illnesses nowadays have been reported to be caused by eating processed meat. Some of these illnesses include heart disease, colon cancer, and high blood pressure. It is because of the presence of chemicals they have that increases the risk of the conditions. Processed meat has been said to contain N-nitroso compounds that are supposed to be cancer-causing. The N-nitroso compounds are made from sodium nitrite, which is used to prevent bacteria and cut food poisoning risks. It also makes the flavor better through rancidification, which means to suppress the oxidation of fat and most of all, to preserve the color of the meat, which is either red or pink. When processed meat products are subjected to high heat, nitrosamines that play significant role illnesses such as bowel cancer forms. One of the oldest methods of meat preservation is smoking. Research shows that smoked meat can contain polycyclic aromatic hydrocarbons, also known as PAHs, which is very harmful to the body. Another reason why it is advisable to keep away from processed meat is that it contains toxic chemical compounds that form when your meat is prepared under high temperatures. These chemical compounds are known as heterocyclic amines. A research was done whereby the heterocyclic amines were given to animals, and they proved that indeed it is cancer-causing. Many studies carried out also showed than when a person frequently consumes well done red meat, they raise their chances of suffering from colon or prostate cancer. For decades, salt has been used as a preservative, but most importantly, its work is to improve the taste of food. When you consume salt excessively, it can easily cause hypertension and other cardiovascular-related illnesses. Processed meat should also be avoided because the amount of salt that goes into their processing is high, and recent studies found out that excessive consumption of salt may cause stomach cancer.

ii. Pizza

Pizza is a food that you should stay away from when on your eating window during intermittent fasting because it has lots of calories and fat that is saturated. It usually leads to fat around the belly. Eating pizza does not add any nutritional value to the body. It only makes you have incredibly high cravings for bad carbohydrates because of getting used to eating starchy foods. When on intermittent fasting, pizza should not be taken because when you consume lots of starch and salt, your body tends to retain water. It will make you gain more weight instead of losing it. Overtime when you feed on pizza, your, body will gain more fat.

iii. Fried chicken.

Fried chicken should be avoided like the plague during intermittent fasting. It is because apart from leading to weight gain, it can lead to significant health issues, including heart problems. A study done showed that consuming fried chicken frequently was associated with many deaths, which were mainly from cardiovascular diseases and cancer. It also shows that those who regularly consume fried chicken are likely to eat fewer vegetables and other healthy foods. They will be craving for sugared beverages like soda, lots of salt, and other unprocessed meats. The bad thing about fried chicken is that it has high levels of salt, calories, and fat, which significantly affect the heart and how it functions daily. The other reason why you should avoid eating fried chicken is that it contains high levels of glycation end products which can easily cause inflammation. The glycation end products are usually are compounds usually formed high temperatures are used for cooking.

iv. Ice cream

Ice cream is one of the things you should stay away from when on your eating window during intermittent fasting because it has very high levels of cholesterol. The downside of the cholesterol in ice cream is that it is known to increase blood cholesterol in your body. This puts you at a high risk of suffering from heart-related illnesses. Another reason why ice cream should be avoided when doing intermittent fasting is that it contains saturated fats. These fats are mostly found in animal products like milk, meat, and even eggs. Just by excessive consumption of ice cream, your blood cholesterol may go up. When it goes up, it increases the risk of suffering from a blockage of the arteries, which will now lead to a stroke or a heart attack. Ice cream also contains too much fat. The body indeed needs fat to produce energy and protect some of the organs in the body, but too much of it will quickly result in cardiovascular disease. Sugar is known to be an empty calorie; therefore, it has no nutrients at all. Ice cream is one of the foods that should not be eaten because it has a lot of sugar, which will lead to weight gain and other heart diseases. When you consume sugar, it can lead to a person who has diabetes because of the quick effect it has on the levels of blood glucose.

v. Artificial sweeteners.

When on intermittent fasting, one of the things you should highly avoid is artificial sweeteners because they lead to weight gain. Studies that were carried out showed that fake sugar caused obesity in both children and grownups. The bad thing about consuming artificial sugars is that it makes your body feel like it needs more calories. That feeling will make you eat even more than you are supposed to. Some of the foods that have artificial sugars are:

- Sweetened yogurt
- Diet drinks especially diet soda
- Protein shakes
- Baked foods and candy
- Pickles
- Salad dressings and
- Ice cream.

People who consumer artificial sugars a lot are said to suffer from metabolic related issues such as excess belly fat, high levels of blood sugar in the body, and abnormal cholesterol levels. All this will eventually put you at a very high risk of stroke and heart disease. When artificial sugar is taken daily, the chance of suffering from cardiovascular disease is high. Insulin is released in the body when artificial sweeteners are consumed without increasing the sugar levels in the blood. Low blood sugar will be caused due to the absorption of sugar in our bloodstream. It makes an artificial sugar consumer suffer from low levels of blood sugar, also known as hypoglycemia. This situation will send a fake signal to our brains that the body needs more sugar to return the blood sugar levels to standard leading to overeating and eventually, obesity. The other reason why artificial sweeteners should be avoided is that it reduces the response of the good bacteria which helps our bodies to maintain optimal health. Our bodies need essential nutrients which help us in fighting disease-causing germs. The microbiota is made up of such bacteria, and the constant use of artificial sugars will decrease it and causing the body to suffer from bacterial imbalance. When the body suffers from bacterial imbalance, it can lead to the inadequate response of the immune system and also lack of proper digestion. A study that was carried out in Europe showed that people who consumed diet beverages that contained artificial sweeteners were more likely to suffer from type 2 diabetes than those who did not. The risk was even more for those who ate artificial sweeteners daily. Artificial sweeteners are just as bad as consuming sugar because their adverse effects are usually the same. The downside of an artificial sweetener is that it is humanmade and thus contains many chemicals. Most of those chemicals are very harmful to the body and can cause very much indigestion and other health issues.

vi. Chocolate

As sweet as it is, the disadvantages of eating chocolate outweigh its nutritional value making it one of the foods to avoid when on intermittent fasting. Chocolate has a very high content of saturated fats and total fats. The number of saturated fat content in chocolate is likely to increase the level of bad cholesterol in your body, putting someone at risk of suffering from heart disease. When you consume dark chocolate, it does not raise your cholesterol levels since it comes from cocoa butter. It not the same as the fat found in milk chocolate. The other reason why during intermittent fasting you should avoid chocolate is because of the high levels of sugar in it. Both sugars in chocolate and other carbohydrates can provide energy just that they have many disadvantages. Chocolate can also cause the tooth to decay and cause heart problems due to its high sugar levels. Another reason why chocolate should be avoided is that it has deficient minerals and vitamin levels.

vii. Doughnuts

Doughnuts are made up of fats and carbohydrates that contain calories of up to 350 per piece. Doughnuts typically have no nutritious benefit on the body because all the used ingredients are refined. Nutrients like fiber are absent in doughnuts due to the refining process. The importance of fiber in the diet is that it reduces cholesterol and sugar levels in the body. Doughnuts are said to also contain trans-fat due to the frying. Eating doughnuts is one of the known causes of obesity. Some of the reasons why you should avoid doughnuts are because just a single serving of doughnut has very high sugar levels. The sugar levels alone will lead to weight gain or even not losing any weight at all when on intermittent fasting. Fats and trans-fats caused by frying will also lead to gain weight due to the high levels of calories present. Doughnuts should be avoided because it increases the levels of blood glucose. The sugar level on the doughnuts, especially those that have fillings will cause your blood sugar to spike because of the glycemic index making the body energy to crash because of the smooth digestion. This will make you feel hungry or crave more easily. Another reason why you should avoid doughnuts when on intermittent fasting is because it can easily cause heart diseases due to the level of saturated fats. The trans-fats found in doughnuts can also make the blood cholesterol and triglycerides, which can easily cause heart disease and even stroke.

viii. Pasta.

Apart from dealing with hunger, pasta has very fewer benefits. During intermittent fasting, pasta is discouraged because it may cause people who are allergic to gluten to react by having mouth ulcers, abdominal bloating depression, and fatigue. In the worst cases, someone who is allergic to gluten and consumes pasta may go into anaphylactic shock. Things like swelling of the throat, being short of breath, vomiting, and blood pressure being low is some of the symptoms of anaphylaxis that may lead to death. Barley, wheat, and rye pasta have gluten that may lead to celiac disease in some people. Celiac is whereby when gluten is swallowed, and it can cause harm to the small intestines.

Pasta is also not suitable during intermittent fasting as it causes fluctuation in the blood sugar levels, and this may lead to a person who has diabetes. People who are gluten intolerant may also suffer from irritable bowel movements. You can also easily take too many calories when having pasta because the chances of overeating are high.

- **What to drink when fasting.**

Starting any lifestyle changes takes time, and it could be confusing at the beginning. After all, you want to do it right. When it comes to intermittent fasting, one of the most common questions asked is: "What can you drink during intermittent fasting?".

Staying hydrated is always essential, but it's even more so during intermittent fasting when your food intake is usually reduced. Roughly 20% of our daily water intake comes from food. Therefore, it is especially important to drink more when you are fasting. One of the side effects of intermittent fasting you might experience is a headache. While it can appear due to several reasons, dehydration is one of the most common ones.

Additionally, a bonus of drinking plenty of liquids while doing intermittent fasting – it can help to overcome the hunger during your fasting period.

To get all the health benefits of Intermittent Fasting such as fat loss, increased metabolic rate, lower blood sugar levels, boost in the immune system, and others, you have to restrict from consuming any caloric food. But you can still consume non-caloric beverages because they do not break your fast and allow you to get all the benefits of fasting.

This is because non-caloric beverages do not cause the release of insulin, and as a consequence, do not interfere with fat burning and autophagy (cellular cleanup).

This would include:

- Water
- Sparkling water
- Mineral water
- Plain black coffee

- Plain tea

But the question is...what exactly can you drink during intermittent fasting to not break your fast?

When fasting, you do not have to start hungry during the entire time. You can take some beverages which will not break your fast. Some of the drinks that can be taken during intermittent fasting are:

i. Coffee

Coffee has zero calories, and drinking; it will not break your fast. Coffee is capable of suppressing hunger, making fasting easily doable. Black coffee cannot break your fast when you take it without milk or cream. The benefits of fasting can also be taken with coffee. Coffee and intermittent fasting can help in reducing inflammation that is chronic as this opens doors to many other diseases in the body. One of the significant inflammation conditions characterized by high cholesterol and excess body fat is metabolic syndrome. Coffee intake usually decreases the risk of metabolic syndrome. Coffee has also been found to improve brain health just as intermittent fasting. Consistent intake of

104

coffee can have been found to reduce the risks of diseases such as Alzheimer's disease. Coffee has also been said to increase autophagy. When on intermittent fasting, the body uses fat to produce energy, which is in the form of ketones. Like we said before, black coffee cannot make you're fast to break. When you put in other additives, you are likely to break your fast and reduce the benefits of fasting. Intermittent fasting can significantly be affected by adding sugar, milk, or even cream in your coffee. Sweetened and coffee that is high in calories should be avoided like the plague during the fasting window. Examples of these types of coffee are cappuccino and lattes. When fasting, making coffee is not a must you can either have it or not. It is a personal choice. As much as coffee does not break a fast, remember it should be taken in moderation and without any additives that have high-calorie content.

ii. Water.

Water is vital as every organ uses it in the body. It is ensuring that you are well-hydrated causes the body not to feel any hunger. Water is an essential drink because apart from making sure you have a regular digestive system, it also ensures that your joints are lubricated and you have a well-regulated body temperature. Research shows that water can also help you burn more calories. When the amount of calories you use up increases, it is called resting energy expenditure. Studies show that, in obese children, the resting energy expenditure increased significantly due to drinking enough water. Studies done on overweight adults showed that drinking 1.5 liters of water daily for a few weeks led to a reduction of fat around the abdomen, weight, and body mass index. Another reason why water is encouraged during intermittent fasting is that it curbs appetite and helps you to eat moderately but still feel full. Thorough research was carried out on adults, and it showed that drinking water before having your meals could cause a person to lose up to 2 kilograms over 12 weeks. Just by drinking water in the morning before having your breakfast, you can significantly reduce the number of calories in that meal by nearly 15%. Water is said to reduce weight since it has zero calories. Parents are also advised to encourage their children to drink water as this will reduce the risk of obesity. It is said that the amount of water intake per day should be 2 liters. Very sporty people hence do lots of exercises may need more water than those who are less active. Water can be found in other foods and drinks as well, such as vegetables, milk, fish, tea, and even fruits. Drinking water through your fasting windows when on intermittent fasting may help you to reduce hunger, headaches, and even prevent someone from having a bad mood. This is because the above symptoms may be caused by mild dehydration. You should also be warned that drinking too much water may cause water toxicity, which is not suitable for your health.

iii. Green tea.

Green tea is said to be one of the healthiest beverages. The antioxidants present in green tea are very advantageous to the body. People who are on intermittent fasting are encouraged to take green tea during the fasting window. It dramatically improves the rate at which fat is lost and also brain activity. Green tea is supported since when you take it, you are guaranteed of improved physical performance. The metabolic rate is also one of the significant improvements which occur by taking green tea. Two studies that were carried out in male adults showed that after taking green tea, the rate at which fat was oxidized was increased by almost 20%. The energy expenditure was also increased. It has also been proven that green tea can protect your brain from diseases such as Alzheimer's and Parkinson's disease. This is possible because it protects your mind for both the short and long term due to the catechin compounds found in green tea that protects neurons in the brain. It will, in turn, protect the brain from neurodegenerative illnesses that leads to Parkinson's disease. Green tea is usually used during intermittent fasting because it has bioactive compounds that are known to improve health. Green tea can also help in the fight against cancer due to the presence of polyphenols, which are very useful in the reduction of inflammation. The catechin, which is also present in green tea helps in the prevention of cell damage. The benefits of green tea are so many. That is why it is advisable to drink it during your fasting period. Another one is that it helps reduce the risk of cancer, such as:

- Colorectal cancer

- Prostate cancer

- Breast cancer.

Another reason why green tea is essential is that it lowers your risk of infection by killing bacteria. It also helps people to avoid cavities in their teeth by killing the harmful bacteria found in the mouth, which is known as streptococcus. It is advisable to take green tea on your fasting window due to its benefit of lowering the risk of diabetes type 2. Just by taking green tea, insulin sensitivity can be significantly reduced and thus reducing the blood sugar levels. Green tea has also been proven to reduce the risk of cardiovascular illnesses. It can also increase the capacity of antioxidant in the blood that prevents the oxidation of LDL. The best benefit of green tea is that it helps in weight loss by boosting the metabolic rate, which eventually decreases body fat. It has also been proven to cause longevity. It is because when you drink it, it lowers your risk of heart disease and cancer that can cut short your life. To become smarter than you are already, all you need is to drink green tea. The key active ingredient is caffeine that blocks the adenosine. It is an inhibitory transmitter of the neurons. From the studies carried out on caffeine, it has been proven that caffeine can improve memory, vigilance, and causes someone to have good moods all day.

iv. Chicken broth

When chicken broth is cooked correctly, it will release nutrients such as magnesium, collagen, gelatin, and calcium. Chicken broth is one of the most amazing foods because even during sickness, they can make you feel better as is a health-boosting drink. It is advisable to drink chicken broth when on intermittent fasting as it helps in reducing inflammation, increases immunity, and protect your gut as well. One of the reasons why chicken broth is advisable during intermittent fasting is that it reduces inflammation and the pains that might be on the joints. This is because it contains glucosamine, which is usually used to cure illnesses in the joint. It reduces joint pain by stimulation of collagen. Chicken broth is so one of the healthy drinks as it promotes healthy digestion by restoring gut health. Gut health is significant because the gut lining is the one that helps to keep dangerous substances from your system. Harmful bacteria and toxins can enter your damage the intestinal walls when they enter your body. When the gut is not healthy or has been damaged, it can cause the intestine to leak. it will then make you susceptible to health issues such as migraines, digestive problems, and even depression.

110

Why the chicken broth is good is because it helps in the restoration of the gut, and improves chronic diarrhea. Another reason why the chicken broth is essential and much advised when on intermittent fasting is because of its capabilities to enhance the skin, hair, and nails. It has a proline that helps in the production of collagen. Collagen has been known for its benefits when it comes to building muscles an excellent skin feel. The reason for taking chicken broth during intermittent fasting is because it has the amino acid known as glycine that can boost anti-inflammatory. The glycine is also essential as it helps in detoxification, which eventually burns fat. The other importance of chicken broth is that it can drastically improve both the repair and growth of bones. This is thanks to the many minerals present in the chicken broth such as phosphor, calcium, and magnesium.

v. Herbal tea.

Herbs, flowers, and roots are some of the ingredients used in making herbal tea. Herbal tea usually has lots of medicinal values which range from relieving stress to treating a cold. Herbal tea can be taken to boost immunity. It is possible because of the presence of vitamins and antioxidants that help in the fight against diseases and infections. Another reason why herbal tea is useful when on the intermittent fasting journey is because it will lower your blood pressure, especially the hibiscus tea. Herbal tea can also be helpful to people who find it hard to sleep. They can benefit from the herbal tea as it calms the mind when taken just before going to bed. One of the herbal teas that reduce stress and anxiety is chamomile tea. It is most comforting as well and might cause mild stimulation in the brain to reduce the feeling of depression. Herbal tea is essential because it has an anti-aging effect. They have antioxidants which research has shown slows down the aging process by reducing the aging of the body cells and preventing them from getting damaged. The herbal tea will make you look and even feel younger, and it will genuinely show on your face and hair. Herbal tea has also been found to improve digestion. Indigestion, bloating, and even vomiting are some of the symptoms that can be cured by taking herbal tea because they cause the breakdown of fat and rapid emptying of the stomach. When you consume herbal tea, it will keep you from taking medicines. For issues like treating cold, it has properties that help in clearing the nasal passage and stops heavy coughs.

vi. Apple juice.

During intermittent fasting, apple juice is one of the essential fluids you can take during your eating window. This is because it has some vital plant proteins that remain when juiced. When apples are made into juice, they usually have a very surprising maximized hydrating quality. Apple juice is essential, especially during intermittent fasting because they are rich in plant proteins such as polyphenols which are mostly found in the apple peel. The plant compounds are vital as they can protect the body against inflammation. Studies show that oxidative damage and inflammation are the major principal factors that cause chronic conditions such as heart disease and cancer. Polyphenols, which are the plant compounds found in apple juice, may be very beneficial when it comes to heart health. Oxidation of harmful cholesterol may be prevented from a buildup in the arteries. This is an essential benefit of apple juice because this build-up may lead to a stroke. The antioxidant boost when apple juice is taken means that the heart is protected against diseases. When on intermittent fasting, apple juice taken during the eating window can be beneficial in that it contains 88% water hence very healthy. The liquid is much recommended because it can cause hydration very fast. It is even better for sick children because they can consume it quickly due to its great taste and the fact that it can speedily hydrate. Extensive research was carried out, and it showed that children who were suffering from diarrhea and vomiting did not fluids delivered via their veins, unlike those that were given electrolytes. Apple juice has also been found to be very important, especially as age starts to catch up as it will support mental health. Unstable molecules in your brain known as free molecules may be damaged, causing the mind not to function at its optimum. Apple juice will protect the brain thanks to the polyphenols and antioxidant activity found in the apple juice.

vii. Soy milk

Soymilk is a nondairy product made from soybeans. Most people, who do not take dairy milk, usually prefer soy milk because it is plant-based. Minerals such as vitamin

D and calcium can be added to the soy milk. One of the reasons why soy milk is advised during intermittent fasting is because it has healthy nutrients and flavonoids that usually protect against inflammation. You can either have soy milk in your smoothie, cereal, or even coffee. Soy milk is the better option if you are doing intermittent fasting, especially if you are lactose intolerant. Milk from cows contains sugars known as lactose, and some people may have trouble digesting it. Soymilk is packed with all the essential amino acids which have many health benefits. It also has the right balance of carbohydrates and fats as well as very high protein levels. Soy milk also has deficient saturated fat, and this will ensure that you do not add weight from it, especially when on intermittent fasting. Soy milk has protective value against heart problems. This is due to the plant compounds found in the liquid that lowers heart-related illnesses. Extensive studies carried out in 2017 showed that women who were overweight and consumed soy milk had the level of bad cholesterol go down by 4%. This alone shows that soy milk can protect against heart disease. Another advantage of soy milk is that it reduces the risk of getting chronic illnesses such as breast and prostate cancer. When on intermittent fasting soy milk is advisable; however, when purchasing, go for the one that is not sweetened.

i. Sea saltwater

When fasting, most nutrients and minerals in your body get depleted fast. That is why it is the importance of having sodium in your meals to help you stay hydrated because the muscle cells will be able to take in water.

For it to work effectively, a person is allowed to add half a teaspoon of sea salt to four liters of water.

ii. Apple cider vinegar

Apple cider is famous during intermittent fasting because it assists the body in the absorption of nutrients and balancing of sugar levels thanks to acetic acid. People with type 2 diabetes or insulin resistance can significantly benefit from vinegar as it will make your blood sugar levels to be healthy. The vinegar will lower blood sugar levels and ensure insulin sensitivity is improved. Another benefit apple cider vinegar is the quick absorption of minerals from food. Apple cider vinegar is essential when fasting because it suppresses the appetite. It is advisable to take apple cider vinegar due to its capability to curb hunger. Extensive research that has been done shows that taking apple cider vinegar can help in the reduction of the body fast and also lower the levels triglycerides in the blood. When you want apple cider vinegar to work well during a fast, you can consume it when you start feeling hungry. Apple cider vinegar has also been found to be very useful in killing harmful bacteria. During the early days, it was used to clean wounds, treat fungus, and other illnesses, including infections of the ears. Vinegar can be used to preserve food whereby, it inhibits bacterial growth in the food. Loss of weight is also another advantage of apple cider vinegar. It is a highly recommended drink when fasting because it can see to it that you consume fewer calories due to the capability of making a person feel full. Apple cider vinegar is perfect when it comes to cardiovascular health. Vinegar consumption can reduce the risk of suffering from heart disease.

iii. Carbonated water.

When carbon dioxide gas is infused with water under pressure, it becomes carbonated water, which is also known as carbonated water. , sodium chloride and other minerals are sometimes added and small amounts to improve the water taste. When a chemical reaction occurs between carbon dioxide and water, carbonic acid is produced. This will help maintain the blood alkalinity. Unlike plain water, when taken, carbonated water may make someone feel fuller for longer hours, and that is why it is recommended during intermittent fasting. Some studies found that carbonated water reduced the chances of constipation. Carbonated or club soda water can improve heart health by decreasing the levels of bad cholesterol. When the water was consumed, it also increased the level of good cholesterol.

- **Drinks discouraged during intermittent fasting**

During intermittent fasting, some drinks are discouraged. This is because they will break the fast and some that have sugar lead to weight gain. Some of the beverages that are not allowed during fasting are:

i. Alcohol

During intermittent fasting, alcohol should never be taken because it can significantly slow down the fat-burning process. Alcohol is also an overeating stimulant, and this can lead to extreme weight gain over time. This is due to its high-calorie level as well. Intermittent fasting is done to reduce weight and inflammation in the body. Alcohol has been proven to promote inflammation making intermittent fasting not have any effect. High levels of inflammation are known to cause illnesses such as cardiovascular disease, type 2diabetes, and cancer. Imbalanced gut bacteria and leaky gut syndrome are one of the diseases caused by inflammation due to excessive drinking. Harmful toxins might be a difficult task for your liver to flash out because of being overwhelmed by alcohol intake. When doing the intermittent fasting, drinking alcohol may cause you to break your fast because it contains calories. Alcohol is also discouraged because it will prevent the process of autophagy from taking place. Autophagy is the process by which dysfunctional proteins are eliminated from the cells to create space for newer cells that are healthier. Autophagy reduces the risk of chronic illnesses such as cancer. The intermittent fasting eating guidelines when doing intermittent fasting is not strict, and as such, alcohol should be taken in moderation.

ii. Soda

Sodas are discouraged during fasting due to the level of empty sugars. A research that was carried out showed that it contains fructose, which is unlikely to lower the hunger levels. People who often take soda are more likely to gain weight faster than those who do not choose soda. When you consume sugar in large amounts, they are eventually turned into fat in the liver. It has been proven that the most common ways to increase fructose in your body are by consuming sugary drinks. Excessive consumption of soda can also lead to fatty liver disease because fat remains in your liver after some have been removed as blood triglycerides. Another reason why you should avoid soda during intermittent fasting is that it increases the accumulation of visceral fat, also known as belly fat. The presence of fructose in the drink is what boosts its ability to accrue fat in other organs as well, which will lead to heart disease diabetes type 2 in the long run. A study that was carried out showed that the people who consumed fructose had substantial amounts of accumulated fats around their belly. However, the ones who consumed fructose only had increased subcutaneous fat. One of the most critical factors that lead to reduced sensitivity in cells is soda intake. Insulin resistance can also be caused by taking soda. It is disadvantageous because the pancreases will be required to make more insulin so as to make even more insulin to eliminate glucose from the bloodstream. This will make insulin levels to go up. Lack of any nutrients is another reason you should stay away from soda when on intermittent fasting. When fasting, we need foods that are rich in minerals, vitamins, and fiber. Soda only adds you calories that make you gain weight instead of losing. Many factors, including leptin resistance can drive weight gain. The hormone leptin is produced by the fat cells in your body for the regulation of calories eaten. Leptin can respond to both responses and adapt to either obesity or starvation. During the fasting period, staying away from sugar is advised as it may give a feeling of pleasure due to the release of dopamine. What this means that consuming a lot of soda and even getting addicted to it is extremely easy. The increase in heart diseases such as blood triglycerides and high levels of blood sugar was also seen in people who consume soda. The consumption of soda as cancer can also cause chronic illnesses such as cancer; obesity, and cardiovascular disease have been seen to go hand in hand. Colorectal cancer recurrence was related to soda and other sweetened beverage intake. When you consume it, the level of fructose in the body rises. Fructose has been known to increase the levels of uric acids, and they crystallize and cause gout.

CHAPTER 6
MYTHS ABOUT INTERMITTENT FASTING

When on intermittent fasting, it is not guaranteed that you will lose weight, but some changes will indeed take place in your body. Below are some of the myths about intermittent fasting that will help you along the way.

Effects on the body

i. Intermittent fasting is starvation.

The difference between intermittent fasting and starvation is huge because deprivation is known to be death or suffering that is caused by hunger. In deprivation, fat stores are usually used up, leaving your body to break down muscle tissue for energy. Skipping a meal for even 48 hours will not make you starve. For your resting metabolic rate to drop, you will have to fast consecutively for over 60 hours. When on intermittent fasting, your tissue and muscle will not be affected in any way since the body will be releasing energy stored as fat.

ii.   It is a must to overeat when on intermittent fasting

It has been said that intermittent fasting makes people eat during their eating window. Sometimes a person may want to pay for the lost calories they would have taken if not for fasting. The truth is, the calories they consume in the food during the eating window is far much less than what they would have taken, were it not for fasting. Intermittent fasting enhances metabolism because it reduces the level of insulin. It is also responsible for human growth hormone improvement.

iii.   You can lose weight by having frequent meals.

Having frequent meals will not boost your metabolic rate. Therefore, it will not affect weight loss in any way. Most people find that smacking a little bit here and there may help them to stay away from eating junk hence reducing their calorie intake.

iv.   You can eat all you want during your eating window and even after you are done fasting.

Intermittent fasting usually acts as a step in a one thousand weight loss journey. If you go back to living an unhealthy lifestyle, the weight will come back and even twice as much. Eating healthy food will help you not to exceed the calories that are expected to maintain the body for the day. It is advisable to have meals that are very balanced like vegetables, fruits, and whole grains. Processed products should be avoided.

v.   You will always be hungry while doing intermittent fasting.

Many people think that when you are on intermittent fasting, you will always be hungry. On the contrary, when your body gets used to it, the hunger pangs will greatly reduce. Studies carried out on people who were suffering from obesity showed that by the second week of intermittent fasting, they could feel very low hunger pangs.

vi.   You have to do intermittent fasting for life once you start.

Intermittent fasting is mostly done to reset your system and kick start your weight loss journey. The beauty about it is that it will keep cravings off. You will not find it as difficult to reject unhealthy foods that will lead to weight gain and chronic illnesses in the long run.

vii.   You will add weight because of not having breakfast.

A lot has been said about breakfast being the most important meal of the day. Contrary to what people believe, skipping breakfast will not make you feel excess hunger and cravings. Breakfast does not affect your weight, but it is an essential meal for school-going children exceptionally if healthy as it is said to help them in performance.

viii.   If you do not eat carbohydrates hourly, your brain will not function.

Some people believe that for your brain to function correctly, it needs carbohydrates, which will be turned to glucose for fueling the brain. What most people do not know is that your body can go through gluconeogenesis, whereby it produces the needed glucose. Dietary fats can help produce ketones even when on a low carbohydrate diet. It will be eaten up by your brain, making it reduces the amount of glucose required.

ix.   You will lose most of your muscles by doing intermittent fasting.

It is not true that when you are on intermittent fasting, your body will use up the muscle to burn fuel. Studies have shown that fasting helps in upholding muscle mass.

x.   Intermittent fasting is not good health-wise.

Fasting has been found to have very many health benefits. It helps to boost immunity, insulin sensitivity helping to prolong the lifespan of a person. Intermittent fasting can also reduce inflammation that will lead to heart diseases later in life. When you fast, you elevate the level of BDNF (brain-derived neurotrophic factor) hormone that protects the brain from suffering from mental illness and even depression.

xi.   Intermittent fasting results are the same for everyone.

All individuals respond differently to intermittent fasting. This is mainly because of the different body structures that make everyone different in their way hence the different results.

Mistakes to avoid when doing intermittent fasting

As we already know, intermittent fasting is used to kick start the weight loss journey, maintain the weight, and has other many health benefits. During the intermittent fasting period, people tend to make some mistakes that will make them not benefit to the maximum doing it. Some of the mistakes we should avoid when fasting is;

i. Not drinking enough water.

Drinking water is vital during fasting because it flushes out toxins which are damaged components of the body. Water and especially sparkling water is also helpful in the intermittent fasting journey. It will help you feel full even when you have not eaten.

ii. Overeating during the eating window

Overeating during intermittent fasting is one of the most natural things to do. This is where many people fail because fasting can leave you very hungry for hours. Unfortunately, as much as intermittent fasting is an essential tool in the weight loss and maintenance journey, you need to eat healthy meals and in moderation. It is even more important to eat healthy when fasting than on regular days to eliminate the possibility of gaining weight and suffering from chronic illnesses.

iii. Starting intermittent fasting too quickly.

One of the biggest reasons why people fail to finish on the intermittent fasting plan is because we exit our routine life too fast to begin. Fasting dramatically affects how we used to eat. It is advisable, to start with, the most straightforward technique of fasting, mainly if you ate after every 3 or 4 hours to make the transition a bit bearable. For beginners, the 12/12 method is usually advised since it may be the easiest.

iv. Restriction of calorie intake during the eating window.

When you have broken your fast, it is advisable to have calories that will see to it that you have not eaten. Not having enough calories will slow down your metabolism. The body will always know when it has had enough. Then, it will release hormones that will signal you that the food you have taken is enough. Undereating usually has some long term disadvantages, such as not being able to lose weight.

v. Fasting and overtraining.

When fasting, it is advisable to do minor exercises. Do not push your body so hard because the production of energy is not so high because of the long hours without food. If you must, do small exercises then with time you will increase the intensity.

vi. Having an obsession over the eating window.

One of the benefits of intermittent fasting is to help you know how to listen to your body more. It will even make it easier to see the difference between when your body is in real hunger. Intermittent fasting will enable you to know when you need to eat, and not the clock dictating the time to eat.

Intermittent fasting is not as easy as it may sound and to help you get through it quickly, we have some tips that will help. Some of the tips are:

i. Ensure you are well hydrated.

When fasting, it is essential to stay hydrated because even the slightest dehydration can cause unwanted symptoms such as headache, fatigue, and feelings of thirst. To help you stay hydrated, medical practitioner advice that you should take at least 2 liters a day. It is advisable to listen to your body and know when it needs more water because the amount of water intake varies from individual to individual. When fasting, dehydration can quickly occur because you get only 30% of the liquid needed by the body from the food we eat.

ii. Do not overeat when breaking a fast.

After a prolonged fast, temptations of overindulging in food are usually very high during the first few days. Overeating will leave you bloated, and you will feel exhausted afterward. If losing weight is your primary goal of doing intermittent fasting, then overeating will surely slow down the process. It may also interfere with the long term benefits of fasting. When you break you're fast, eat normally, and continue with your daily routine.

iii. Keep your fasting periods short.

The duration of fasting usually depends on an individual. For beginners taking shorter fasting, periods may be the best option. However, people who have done fasting for some time may go for long periods with some even going for up to 48 hours. More extended fasting periods can sometimes have a negative effect as some people get easily irritable, lack of focus, and even fainting. Longer fasts may also cause dehydration and lack of energy. These side effects can be evaded by sticking to fasting periods that are a bit shorter. Medical opinion is vital before starting a 72 hour fast.

iv. Do not fast if you feel sick.

When doing intermittent fasting, some of the symptoms that you will face are hunger, being easily irritable, and feeling tired. When you feel unwell, kindly consider stopping the fast and seek medical advice. Also, ensure that you do not fast for more than 24 hours and that you always have a snack with you. Some of the healthy snacks are nuts which should be eaten in moderation as well.

v. Ensure you do very mild exercises.

When fasting, people go through different experiences, so it is not unusual to find other people doing high-intensity exercises. When you are just starting to fast, it is ok to do mild exercises, and if you feel your body can not take it, it is ok to stop. Some of the low-intensity activities include walking, yoga, and even housework.

vi. Feed on whole meal foods during non-fasting days.

Intermittent fasting is usually abstaining from food for specified periods to lose weight and have other health benefits. It is therefore crucial that when not fasting, you should feed on healthy wholemeal foods. Examples of such foods are fish, eggs, vegetables, and lean meat since they have very many health benefits.

vii. Ensure your meals have lots of proteins.

Having enough proteins in your meals is vital as they protect you from being in a calorie deficit. The downside of being in a calorie deficit is that apart from losing fat, it can lead to loss of muscle. You are also allowed to feed on small portions of proteins during your fast days. It will help in the reduction of hunger and reduce the number of side effects brought about by fasting.

viii. Use supplements.

When fasting, getting essential nutrients is not easy. This makes it a bit hard to reach your nutritional value because of the reduced calorie intake. Vitamin B12, iron, and calcium are some of the critical nutrients that people who are on weight-loss diets lack. For the prevention of deficiencies, those who are doing intermittent fasting should think about using the multivitamin to prevent the body from lacking essential nutrients.

ix. Meditate

Doing intermittent fasting is not easy, especially if you are not busy and bored. This might lead you into temptations of eating, thus breaking your fast. Meditation can keep your mind occupied and help in to destruct you from hunger without using too much energy. Another way that you can use to keep your mind busy without using too much power is by taking a walk or reading a book.

CHAPTER 7
HOW TO START INTERMITTENT FASTING

The only thing you should decide before you start is which type of schedule are you planning to follow. And before you make this decision, it is essential to understand the various types of Intermittent Fasting. That's how you will find the one that works the best for you and fits your unique lifestyle.

It takes more time to learn about intermittent fasting for women than it takes to start it!

The best way to get started is to choose one method and give it a try. Getting started is simple. Chances are you've already done many intermittent fasting days before. Many of us instinctively eat this way, skipping morning or evening meals -not always on purpose but because we're not hungry or full from eating a more substantial meal in the afternoon.

The easiest way to get started is to choose one of the intermittent fasting methods above and give it a go. However, you don't need to follow a structured plan necessarily. An alternative is to fast whenever it suits you. Skipping meals from time to time when you don't feel hungry or don't have time to cook can work as well.

It doesn't matter which type of fast you choose. The most important thing is to find a method that works best for you and your lifestyle. Just remember to eat a healthy diet during your non-fasting periods. Only because you are fasting, it doesn't mean you can eat a crappy diet the rest of the time and still expect to get weight loss and health results from your fast.

For your convenience, here are the most popular Intermittent Fasting Schedules.

Intermittent Fasting 16/8

How: Fast for 16 h and Eat 8 h

By following this 16/8 Intermittent Fasting Schedule, you fast for 16 hours and restrict your eating to an 8-hour eating window.

It is really up to you which 16 out of 24 hours you will decide to restrict yourself from eating. You can choose to have an eating window from 8 am to 4 pm, 10 am to 6 pm, noon to 8 pm or any other schedule, as long as it is 16h of continuous non-eating.

The majority of the people who follow this schedule, choose to skip breakfast rather than dinner, but different people have different life rhythms.

What's great, that out of 16h, you'll probably be sleeping at least 7-8 of them, so we're just talking about 9-8h of fasting each day.

It's also worth noting that we believe Intermittent Fasting 16/8 method is the most sustainable and easiest to start with.

How: Fast for 18 h and Eat 6 h

Almost identical to the one above, if you choose the 18/6 Intermittent Fasting Schedule, you should fast for 18 hours and restrict your eating to a 6-hour eating window.

It's just two more hours of fasting daily, but for a beginner faster, these 2 hours can make all the difference.

That's why we recommend starting with 16/8 for at least a month until moving to 18/6 because you'll have a much more enjoyable start, and that's a crucial element between quitting and not.

Slow and steady wins the race – take it easy and listen to your body before going extreme.

Intermittent Fasting 5:2 A.K.A The Fast Diet

How: 2 days per week restrict calories to 500-600, 5 days per week eat normally

5:2 Intermittent Fasting lets you eat regularly 5 days per week and restricts your calorie intake to 500-600 per day during the other 2 days. When choosing your fasting days, keep in mind that there should be at least one regular eating day in between.

Please note that your results depend on what you eat during the 5 days of non-fasting, thus stick to the nutritious and whole diet throughout for max results.

Intermittent Fasting 20/4 A.K.A. Warrior Diet

How: Fast for 20 h and Eat for 4h.

In contrast to other methods, while following the 20/4 Intermittent Fasting Schedule, you are allowed to eat some raw fruits and vegetables and some lean protein during the 20 hr fast period.

This schedule is based on the idea that our ancestors spent their days hunting and gathering and would then feast at night. Therefore the 4-hour eating window shall be in the evening, and you should follow a particular order of eating specific food groups: starting with vegetables, proteins and fat, and eating carbs only if you are still hungry.

Omad Fasting - One Meal A Day A.K.A 23 /1

How: Fast for 23h and eat once a day

Another popular fasting schedule is called one-meal-a-day (OMAD).

It is precisely what it sounds like – you choose a time in a day that is the most suitable for you to have your on and only meal of the day.

I know what you're thinking – isn't that almost starving? And yes, you are right – OMAD diet shouldn't be done without thought on how to get at least 1200 calories during that one meal.

Thus if you choose this schedule – make sure your meal is a hearty and nutritious one.

24 Hr Fast A.K.A. Eat Stop Eat

How: Fast for 24 h 1-2 times a week

While following 24 hours fast (popularized by Eat Stop Eat method, you should fast for 24 hours 1-2 days a week and normally eat on other days, that way you should reduce overall calorie intake by ca 10%, and hence lose weight.

Circadian Rhythm Fasting

How: Start fasting when the sun goes down and start eating when the sun goes up

You might have heard that our bodies have been designed to follow Circadian rhythm – an internal clock that runs 24h each day and regulates our energy levels based on the rhythm of the day and night.

Thus if you follow Circadian Rhythm fasting, you would allow daylight to decide your hours.

As soon as the sun is up – your eating window starts. As soon as it is down and it gets dark – you should start your fasting.

The only downside of it is that the success of it depends on where you live. In some places on our Planet Earth-like northern Norway, the sun never sets for 76 days a year.

Extended A.K.A Prolonged Fastings

How: Fast for more than 24 hours once a month

As mentioned before, extended or prolonged fasting usually means anything between 24 and 96 hours of fasting.

It is not recommended to do it more often than once a month, and anything above 48-72h of fasting should be done under the doctor's supervision.

Yes, there are lots of people who don't follow this recommendation, and nothing happens, but it is risky.

Recommended Intermittent Fasting Schedule For Women

Everyone's body is different, so there is no one size fits all approach to intermittent fasting.

Generally speaking, though, women should take a more gentle approach to fast than the average man.

Here are some of the types of intermittent fasting women are most successful with:

Crescendo Method: Fast for 12-16 hours two to three days per week. Fasting days should always be non-consecutive and spaced out as evenly as possible.

Eat-Stop-Eat: Fast for 24-hour periods once or twice a week. If you want to try this method, start with 14-hour fasts and work your way up to 24 hours. During the other days, just eat responsibly.

5:2 Diet: Eat what you want with this method (within reason, of course!) 5 days a week, and then for two non-consecutive days, eat 25% of your regular calorie allotment. About 500 calories for women, 600 for men.

16/8 Method: Fast for 16 hours, eat for 8 hours. This method works for those that don't usually get hungry in the morning, and most of the fasting will be spent sleeping. Try starting with a 14-hour fast period and build up to 16 hours.

Modified Alternate Day Fasting: Fast every other day. Eat about 500 calories (20-25% of your usual daily calorie amount) on your fasting day, and usually eat on non-fasting days.

Remember that during your eating periods, you are not restricting calories. But also remember that you need to make good choices and eat a healthy diet to get the most out of intermittent fasting for women. You can't outrun a bad diet and you can't out-fast a bad diet either!

Safety Of Intermittent Fasting

Modified versions of intermittent fasting should be safe for most women. That said, always be safe when trying any new health routine.

If you have a medical condition, you should talk to your doctor before starting any diet or health routine.

Seek medical advice before trying intermittent fasting if you are a woman who:

- Is underweight.
- Is pregnant, breastfeeding, or trying to become pregnant.

- Hase a history of missed periods or fertility problems.
- Has a history of eating disorders.
- Has diabetes or problems with low blood sugar.

Intermittent Fasting Side Effects

Most intermittent fasting side effects are minor and go away once you've been fasting for a while.

Some common side effects that you may experience when you first start are:

- Hunger
- Cravings
- Headaches
- Low Energy
- Irritability
- Heartburn
- Feeling Cold
- Overeating

Anytime you are starting a new routine, ease your body into it. If you are used to eating six meals a day, don't suddenly start eating one meal a day. Listen to your body and cut your fast short if you feel you need to.

How Intermittent Fasting Affects Women Differently Than Men

Calorie restriction can inhibit the production of female sex hormones causing irregular periods, infertility, and hormonal imbalances. This is why it's essential that women who intermittent fast do not do it for caloric restriction but the health and wellness aspect.

When women restrict their calories, their metabolism slows down, hormones go out of balance, and the body cannot function at their optimal levels.

So, if you're a woman that's restricting her calories and intermittent fasting, you're doing your body more harm than good and losing the benefits of intermittent fasting.

Intermittent fasting can be beneficial for women when incorporated in a weight loss program, given that the body continues to receive the nutrition it needs.

It's important to know that intermittent fasting can have different effects on women of different ages.

If you are post-menopausal, intermittent fasting won't be such a risk to your overall health, albeit pre-menopausal women are more likely to experience poor outcomes with extreme or moderate forms of intermittent fasting — emphasis on the absolute or moderate.

CHAPTER 8

HACKS OF SUCCESSFUL INTERMITTENT FASTING

Like we have seen in the topics above, intermittent fasting is not easy. We need support as much as possible and anything that can make your journey easier. Below are some of the hacks that will make your journey smooth.

HACKS

i. Decide on your fasting window.

Intermittent fasting is not a strict time-based diet. This means that you can choose the number of hours to fast and when to fast either day or night. The fasting and eating window periods are not a must to be the same every day.

ii. Ensure you get enough sleep.

When you get enough sleep, you become healthier, and your overall well-being is guaranteed. When we sleep, the body operates certain functions in the body that helps burn calories and improves the metabolic rate.

iii. Eat healthy Avoid eating anything you want after a fast.

Healthy meals should be your focus. They will help you get the required nutrients like vitamins, which will give you more energy during the fasting period.

iv. Drink more water.

One of the best decisions you can make during a fast is to drink water. It will keep your body hydrated and taking water before meals can significantly reduce appetite.

v. Start small.

If you have never tried it before, there is no way you start fasting and go for a whole 48 hours without a meal. For beginners, you can start by having your food at 8 pm, for example, and having nothing again until 8 am the next day. It will be easier since sleep is incorporated in your eating window.

vi. Avoid stress.

Intermittent might be hard to do if you are stressed. This is because stress can trigger an overindulgence of food to some people. It is also easier to feed on junk when stressed to feel better. That's why when on intermittent fasting, you are advised to avoid if not control your stress levels.

vii. Be disciplined.

Remember that fasting means the abstinence of food until a particular time. When fasting, be true to yourself and avoid eating before the stipulated time. It will ensure that you lose maximum weight and benefit health-wise from intermittent fasting.

viii. Keep off flavored drinks.

Most flavored drink says that they are low in sugar, but in the real sense, they are not. Flavored drinks contain artificial sweeteners, which will affect your health negatively. They will also increase your appetite, causing you to overeat, and this will make you gain weight instead of losing.

ix. Find something to do when fasting.

It is said that an idle mind is the devil's workshop. When you are on intermittent fasting and not busy, you will be thinking about food, and this will make you break your fast before the stipulated time. You can keep yourself busy by running errands, listening to music, or even taking a walk in the park.

x. Exercising

Exercise can be done when fasting, but it is not a must. Mild exercises can be done even at home. By exercising, you will build your muscle strength, and your body fat will burn faster.

How intermittent fasting affect women and men

As we now know, intermittent fasting is the abstinence from food. It dramatically affects our bodies both and positively and negatively. When on intermittent fasting, the females may suffer from irregular periods and hormonal imbalance because of the calorie inhibition of the sex hormones. Some women also experience disturbances on their metabolism and can even suffer from early menopause. When they fast, women experience out of balance hormones. That leads to a lack of optimal body function, but the good news is that it also has many benefits in both men and women. One of the advantages is that it protects a person from diabetes. This is made possible because intermittent fasting reduces insulin levels and insulin resistance. Intermittent fasting also caused weight loss in men and women. During your eating window, the number of calories you consume will determine the weight you lose. Intermittent fasting can also reduce the chances of heart disease in

155

women and men and has been proved to suppress appetite. This will keep you from eating on meals that are unhealthy and will also let your body know when you are starving. Psychological health is also one of the benefits of fasting. A study that was carried out showed that women were no longer as depressed as they were before they started fasting. Another effect of intermittent fasting on men and women is that in both, their muscle mass was also retained. When they were done fasting, it helped them in burning of more fat even when resting. In men, a study showed that intermittent fasting did not worsen the control of blood sugar like the one it did in women. The female body is usually very delicate when it comes to the restriction of calories. Unlike in the male body; therefore, In women, the hypothalamus is affected when you fast more frequently affecting the hormones that are used to release the reproductive hormones. Intermittent fasting can cause infertility in women. It happens when the follicle-stimulating and luteinizing hormones fail to communicate with gonadotropin hormone. Thorough research carried out in the female rats showed that six months of intermittent fasting caused their ovaries to reduce in size. As for men, they are luckier than women when it comes to intermittent fasting because of their reproductive functions are not connected to their metabolic function. Intermittent fasting is also beneficial in men since it has been proven to increase testosterone levels. In both men and women, fasting was found to help focus. In both men and women, intermittent fasting has been shown to break an addiction. It is because it teaches one to be disciplined and follow the rules to the later to achieve great results such as weight loss and cardiovascular health. For men and women who hate exercising, intermittent fasting can be used to kick off weight loss journey and eventually a healthy life.

CHAPTER 9

CAN INTERMITTENT FASTING EXTEND A WOMAN'S FERTILITY?

If intermittent fasting can extend female fertility is a topic that has been asked for a while, but recent studies that were carried out have now shed light on this question. It is no secret that aging causes the reduction of quality and quantity of eggs. The studies were carried out in mice whereby their calorie intake was reduced by 40%. It had significantly improved their egg quality and found out that just a few of their eggs contained abnormal chromosomes when they got to their reproductive years. This is not the same as their counterparts that were allowed to eat as much as they wanted. It is the abnormalities in eggs that usually causes congenital disabilities and raises the risk of having miscarriages. The study further showed that mice that underwent intermittent fasting were able to produce more eggs than the mice that ate as they liked. Restriction of calories also increased the survival of the offspring after birth and also prolonged their reproductive life span. This study concluded that when you manipulate nutrition, you can adjust the signal pathways. Another study was carried out on worms showed that during intermittent fasting, they put reproduction on hold. It helped them to terminate the sex cells that existed to be able to generate healthy eggs. The lifespan of the worms that underwent the process above was greatly extended. Human beings may go through the same process, but tests are yet to be done. The PPAR gamma is the protein that scientists say might do the job of controlling the rate at which ovulation occurs. The studies are also not clear about the amount of calorie restriction that will be needed to turn on such systems in human beings. A lot of fertility problems could be solved if only the identification and manipulation of signaling molecules could be done. This could even extend the reproductive life span of a woman. Fasting has been said to improve chances of couples that have been trying to conceive through in vitro fertilization but were never successful. Fertility specialists found out that intermittent fasting can alkalize the blood system, removes the synthetic hormones, and cleanse the liver. They also said that when you fast, the body's natural hormone process is rebooted. The calorie intake of people who take the time or find it hard to conceive is usually evaluated. If it is high, with the help of a nutritionist, they are started on intermittent fasting. This will not only get rid of toxins in the patient's body, but it will also help them to get closer to their required Body mass index. Intermittent fasting will cause the rebalancing of hormones, and the liver will metabolize any excess hormones. Fasting will also cause the regeneration of all organs in the body, and issues like inflammation are reduced. It will also boost the immune system and cause the nervous system to be to rest hence making the reproductive system prepared for conception. In males, intermittent fasting can greatly increase the sperm count from men who suffer from fertility issues. It can also boost the levels of testosterone hormones in men who do not suffer from fertility issues.

Intermittent fasting for pregnant women

Intermittent fasting is whereby you voluntarily stay away from food for hours at a time and choose to eat at certain times. Different individuals choose intermittent fasting

160

for various reasons, but the most popular ideas are weight loss and for health benefits. During pregnancy, most women suffer from nausea, and you might start to dislike some foods, usually due to the shifts that happen to hormones that will help in sustaining the pregnancy. When pregnant, the pancreas will grow to produce more insulin. During the first trimester, being nauseous all the time may make it hard for you to overeat on one sitting. Many pregnant women will want to feed on carbohydrates, which will leave you hungry after a short while. It makes intermittent fasting almost impossible due to the number of times you will snack due to hunger. During the second trimester, for most people by now, nausea will have reduced. It can only mean that you can go back to eating a more healthy diet which has fewer carbohydrates and more vegetables and proteins. It will make you stay fuller for longer hours. Fasting while pregnant is not advisable because, during this period, all you need to do is ensure that your micronutrient needs are met. Some pregnant women can go through with fasting without any issue, which is okay. What is not allowed is if you are forcing yourself to fast even though your body is sending hunger signals. The third trimester is where your body's demand for macronutrients is high. When you sleep at night, your body will naturally fast. Therefore, it is not advisable to force your body to go without food because either way, the body typically gains weight. Caution should be applied even though you are advised to eat frequently because overeating junk can cause gestational diabetes, fetal macrosomia, or even preeclampsia. Fasting also is not good when pregnant because the fetus needs nutrients that will support its well-being in the tummy. Fasting is discouraged because when pregnant, the need for protein will be high; hence cannot be met in an 8-hour eating window.

The growing fetus makes the needs for calories and macronutrients high as well and almost impossible to be met in an 8-hour eating window. Your body will also go through some major changes which are hormonally induced because your boy wants to grow a baby. Intermittent fasting should be the last thing on your mind as your total focus should be on the growing fetus.

Extensive research that was carried out on breastfeeding mums showed that short term fasting would not decrease your milk supply. Dehydration is what might cause the decrease in milk. Mothers with babies who are below five months were studied. It was clear that fasting does not affect breast milk or the growth of the baby through what happens is that some essential nutrients in breast milk will reduce. One of the downsides of fasting when breastfeeding is that, you can get dehydrated very fast. This will, in turn, lead to the reduction of breast milk supply and for some mothers it can be extremely difficult to get their milk supply back up. Some of the tips that a breastfeeding mother can use are:

Ensure your water intake is high.

For you to maintain milk supply, you need to drink water. This will help to keep you hydrated and reduce hunger pangs.

Consumption of healthy meals.

Eating healthy meals such as vegetables, proteins, and healthy fats such as avocado and nuts will help you go through intermittent fasting smoothly. It will help in the reduction of cravings, and you will only eat healthy foods that will make you feel fuller for longer.

Always start small.

More often than not, after giving birth, all women think about is losing the baby fat. Intermittent fasting may help you shed off a few kilos. Remember, even when in the quest for losing weight, your number one priority should be you and the baby's health. For you to keep your milk supply constant, start small by trying the 12-hour fasting, which is usually the easiest. From there, you can increase your fasting hours gradually.

Be keen and listen to your body.

There is a difference between real hunger, and your body wants to eat. If you are keen enough, you will know whether it's real hunger or if you wish to eat. It is also advisable to pay attention to what triggers your emotions making it easy for you to eat. Make sure you are keen to understand how what you eat affects your body negatively.

Have meal plans.

When on intermittent fasting, it is advisable to have a meal plan. Usually, it is effortless to eat unhealthy foods. Due to hunger, you will eat anything you find, which is less likely to be a balanced diet. Planning will see to it that you eat healthy at all times.

Avoid over-exercising.

Never overdo your exercises. When breastfeeding and on intermittent fasting, it is advisable to stay away from tough workouts. You should increase your intensity as you go because due to starvation, the body does not have a lot of energy. Only mild exercises such as walking and house chores should be done.

Ensure you consume proteins and fiber in all meals.

The advantage of having meals with lots of fiber and proteins is that you will feel fuller for more extended hours, making you avoid overeating or consuming unhealthy foods.

CHAPTER 10
THE FASTING AND HORMONE CONNECTION

To put it simply, intermittent fasting can cause hormonal imbalance in women if it's not done correctly. Women are extremely sensitive to signals of starvation, and if the body senses that it is being starved, it will ramp up production of the hunger hormones leptin and ghrelin.

So when women experience insatiable hunger after under-eating, they are experiencing the increased production of these hormones. It's the female body's way of protecting a potential fetus — even when a woman is not pregnant.

Of course, though, many women ignore these hunger cues causing the signals to get even louder. Or, worse, we try to ignore them, then fail and binge later, then follow that up with under-eating and starvation again. And guess what? That vicious cycle can throw your hormones out of whack and even halt ovulation.

In animal studies, after two weeks of intermittent fasting, female rats stopped having menstrual cycles, and their ovaries shrunk while experiencing more insomnia than their male counterparts (though the male rats did experience lower testosterone production).

Unfortunately, there are very few human studies looking at the differences between intermittent fasting for men and women. Still, the animal studies confirm our suspicion: Intermittent fasting for long periods can sometimes throw off a woman's hormonal balance, cause fertility problems and exacerbate eating disorders like anorexia, bulimia, and binge eating disorder.

Insulin

Insulin is one of the main hormones involved in fat metabolism. It tells your body to store fat and also stops your body from breaking fat down.

Having chronically high levels of insulin can make it much harder to lose weight. High levels of insulin have also been linked to diseases like obesity, type 2 diabetes, heart disease, and cancer.

Intermittent fasting is just as effective as calorie-restricted diets for lowering your insulin levels.

This eating style could reduce fasting insulin levels by 20–31%.

If you have insulin resistance, pre-diabetes, Type 2 Diabetes, or any glucose metabolism issues, they need to be addressed right away if you want to lose weight.

And the 3-Week Intermittent Fasting Diet focuses on the #1 hormone that affects your ability to lose stubborn weight, insulin.

Human Growth Hormone (HGH)

HGH is one of the most underrated weight loss hormones, especially for women.

Girl, let me dish on why HGH is a hormone you should pay attention to.

Fasting can cause a rise in blood levels of human growth hormone, an essential hormone for promoting fat loss.

Some studies have shown that in men, levels of human growth hormone may increase by as much as five-fold while fasting.

Increases in blood levels of human growth hormone not only promote fat burning, but they also preserve muscle mass and have other benefits.

However, women don't always experience the same benefits from fasting as men. And here is the reason.

Women shouldn't fast the same as men.

Since a woman's hormonal system is much more delicate than a man's, you need to fast strategically.

Enter "metabolic fasting."

Metabolic fasting doesn't just allow you to skip meals and fast in a normal sense.

Metabolic fasting addresses why food quality, macro balancing, carb pairing, food combining, and exercise are essential for losing weight and boosting HGH (and other fat-burning hormones).

Norepinephrine

Norepinephrine, a stress hormone that improves alertness and attention, is involved in the "fight or flight" response.

It has a variety of other effects on your body, one of which is telling your body's fat cells to release fatty acids.

Increases in norepinephrine generally lead to more significant amounts of fat being available for your body to burn.

Fasting leads to a rise in the amount of norepinephrine in your bloodstream.

Women don't respond the same way men do when it comes to "traditional" intermittent fasting.

It's not fair. But that doesn't mean you can't get all of the benefits of intermittent fasting.

You just need to "fast outside of the box."

See, most people who start intermittent fasting, end up right where they end up with any diet.

They lose a bunch of weight, feel great, but then. The weight starts creeping back. Then you start up again and repeat the vicious cycle of losing weight, gaining weight, losing weight, and gaining it back.

See, most Intermitent fast experts just tell you to fast a day or a certain number of hours, then eat whatever you want when you aren't fasting.

This approach might make you happy, but it's not helping your hormones.

And hormones are my wheelhouse!

To prevent regaining the weight, you need to address hormones, metabolism, and health.

Get healthy to lose weight, NOT the other way around.

Metabolic fasting is my solution to harmful intermittent fasting programs that promise results that just don't last.

Fasting And Female Hormones

In the grand scheme of your life's health decisions, experimenting with IF seems tiny, right? Unfortunately — for some women, at least — it looks like small decisions can have significant impacts.

It turns out that the hormones regulating key functions like ovulation are incredibly sensitive to your energy intake.

In both men and women, the hypothalamic-pituitary-gonadal (HPG) axis — the cooperative functioning of three endocrine glands — acts a bit like an air traffic controller.

- First, the hypothalamus releases gonadotropin-releasing hormone (GnRH).
- This tells the pituitary to release luteinizing hormone (LH) and follicular stimulating hormone (FSH).
- LH and FSH then act on the gonads (a.k.a. testes or ovaries).

"In women, this triggers the production of estrogen and progesterone — which we need to release a mature egg (ovulation) and to support a pregnancy."

"In men, this triggers the production of testosterone and sperm production."

Because this chain of reactions happens on a particular, regular cycle in women, GnRH pulses must be very precisely timed, or everything can get out of whack.

GnRH pulses seem to be very sensitive to environmental factors and can be thrown off by fasting.

Even short-term fasting (say, three days) alters hormonal pulses in some women.

There's even some evidence that missing a single regular meal (while of course not constituting an emergency es are ready to quickly respond to the change in energy intake if it continues.

Maybe this is why certain women do just fine with IF while others run into problems. by itself) can start to put us on alert, perking up our antennae, so our body.

Why does Intermittent Fast affect women's hormones more than men's?

This might have something to do with kisspeptin, a protein-like molecule that neurons use to communicate with each other (and get important stuff done).

Kisspeptin stimulates GnRH production in both sexes, and we know that it's susceptible to leptin, insulin, and ghrelin — hormones that regulate and react to hunger and satiety.

Interestingly, females mammals have more kisspeptin than males. More kisspeptin neurons may mean higher sensitivity to changes in energy balance.

This may be one reason why fasting more readily causes women's kisspeptin production to dip, tossing their GnRH off-kilter.

CHAPTER 11
WHICH DIET TO CHOOSE?

These Intermittent Fasting Meal Plans are created to support your weight goals and are equally effective no matter which diet you chose.

1. Keto Meal Plan is based on a 25% protein, 5% carbohydrates, and 70% fat macronutrient breakdown. It is tailored for those that are looking to burn fat more effectively by putting the body into a metabolic state called ketosis.

   What Is Keto Diet?

The ketogenic diet is a low-carb, moderate in protein and a high-fat diet, which helps you burn fat more effectively. Ketogenic diet plan involves drastically reducing carb intake and replacing it with fat to put the body into a metabolic state called ketosis.

The Intermittent Fasting Keto Meal Plan is based on a low-carb Keto diet, with 25% protein, 5% carbohydrates, and 70% fat macronutrient distribution.

2. Vegan Keto Meal plan is based on a vegan low carb diet with max daily net carbs of 50g to promote ketosis.

What Is Vegan Keto Diet?

The ketogenic diet is a low-carb, moderate in protein and a high-fat diet, which helps you burn fat more effectively. Ketogenic diet plan involves drastically reducing carb intake and replacing it with fat to put the body into a metabolic state called ketosis. Combined with Intermittent Fasting, it's a super useful weight-loss tool.

The Vegan Keto Meal Plan is based on a low-carb vegan keto diet, with max net carbs of 50g a day to reach Ketosis.

Vegan keto meal plan has a slightly higher amount of carbohydrates as compared to our regular keto plan to ensure as a vegan, you get enough fiber and protein through a greater variety of natural food sources.

3. Regular Intermittent Fasting Meal Plan emphasizes macronutrient balance with a particular emphasis on protein to promote satiety and weight management (30% protein, 40% carbohydrates, and 30% fat).

What Is Regular Intermittent Fasting?

The Intermittent Fasting regular-omnivore meal plan is designed to support a healthy, balanced, and versatile diet. Proteins are high in this meal plan to promote healthy weight management and reduce appetite.

It supports consuming two meals and one snack a day and is based on 30% protein, 40% carbohydrates, and 30% fat macronutrient distribution.

4. Vegetarian Meal Plan is based on a lacto-vegetarian diet with 30% protein, 40% carbohydrates, and 30% fat macronutrient distribution.

What Is Vegetarian Diet Meal Plan?

The vegetarian diet plan devoids animal products such as meat, poultry, fish, seafood, and any foods containing ingredients derived from these products.

Our vegetarian meal plan is based on a Lacto-Vegetarian diet, which allows the usage of dairy but no eggs.

To support satiety and healthy weight management, vegetarian protein sources have been emphasized, such as dairy, whole grains, vegetables, fruits, and calcium-rich foods.

5. Vegan Meal Plan contains only foods made from plants and has a macronutrient distribution of 20% protein, 40% carbohydrates, and 40% fat.

What Is Vegan Diet?

Vegan diet devoids any animal products and any foods containing ingredients derived from animals.

The vegan meal plan, a.k.a. Plant-based diet meal plan supports a healthy, balanced, and versatile vegan diet, and is designed to be used in combination with Intermittent Fasting.

To support satiety and weight management, plant-based proteins such as legumes, high protein nuts, seeds, and grains are emphasized in all our vegan meals across the plan.

6. Paleo Meal Plan focuses on a 'caveman' diet that includes lean meats, fish, fruits, veggies, nuts and seeds, and foods. It is based on a 30% protein, 40% carbohydrates, and 30% fat macronutrient distribution.

What Is Paleo Diet?

Paleo diet, also called the Paleolithic diet, Stone Age diet, caveman diet or hunter-gatherer diet is based on foods that back in time was obtained by hunting and gathering, such as lean meats, fish, fruits, vegetables, nuts, and seeds. It eliminates dairy products, legumes, grains, sugar, and processed food.

By switching 'back' to the way our ancestors were eating, you can lose weight, reduce inflammations, the risk for heart disease, cholesterol, blood pressure, and improve overall health.

Despite being slightly more sensitive to Intermittent Fasting than men, women can still practice time-restricted eating and experience all the intermittent fasting benefits, including weight loss.

However, there are some essential factors to take into account before you embark on the Intermittent Fasting journey.

Caloric Intake

With fewer hours to consume food, you will likely be consuming fewer calories, and as learned earlier, female bodies are more sensitive to caloric restriction.

Therefore it is essential to take a more relaxed approach to intermittent fasting, start slow and listen to your body.

If you experience any of the severe side effects like a missed period or constant fatigue, take a break and consult with your doctor. A professional will be

182

able to advise the best approach for your unique situation or recommend alternative means to reach your weight loss or diet goals.

Diet Quality

Intermittent fasting should by no means be a way out of a bad diet.

Nutritional deficiencies when not getting enough macronutrients (carbs, protein, and fats) or micronutrients (vitamins and minerals) are more common among women, particularly young women during childbearing age, and is linked with poor diet choices. Having a nutritious, balanced diet is the key when doing intermittent fasting to avoid most side effects of fasting.

Weight And Body Mass Index (BMI)

Studies show that it is essential to make a distinction between different body weights when looking at side effects and benefits of Intermittent Fasting.

Overweight and obese women show significant improvements with Intermittent Fasting, while women with healthy weight did not experience the same across-the-board metabolic benefits.

Underweight women should be particularly careful when doing intermittent fasting. Even if you don't need to lose weight, you can still enjoy other benefits of Fasting, such as cell regeneration, improved energy levels, and reduced blood sugar levels. But, it's crucial to make sure you have a nutritious diet and sufficient caloric intake to avoid intermittent fasting side effects.

For a generally healthy person, it is okay to start beginner-friendly intermittent fasting methods like intermittent fasting 16/8 on their own.

However, you should consult with your doctor if you:

- Are underweight or struggling with weight gain. Your eating window will be a lot shorter, which means it will be harder to consume the same amount or more calories than normal.
- Are pregnant or breastfeeding. You should be more cautious with your diet and lifestyle during this time.
- Are under 18 years old. Effects of intermittent fasting during periods of rapid growth, such as for children and teenagers, are not studied enough. Therefore, you should be cautious about it.
- Have suffered from an eating disorder. Restricting times of eating will increase the risk of falling back into old habits during an eating disorder.
- Have type 1 diabetes. Intermittent fasting increases sensitivity to insulin. Therefore it may affect how much insulin medication you need.

Remember, as a woman; it's crucial to ease into Intermittent Fasting slowly.

Sudden diet and lifestyle changes might come with many side effects like loss of energy, headache, trouble sleeping, rapid mood swings, and others.

If you are planning on starting the most popular Intermittent Fasting method, 16/8 let your body adapt to the new eating pattern by starting with a 12/12 schedule. It would mean 12 hours of fasting and a 12-hour eating window. Slowly increase your fasting window as the days go by until you have reached your desired Intermittent Fasting schedule.

CHAPTER 12

INTERMITTENT FASTING TIPS AND TRICKS

Here's a quick overview of some of the key concepts of Intermittent Fast and what to keep in mind if you want to try it.

First, decide if it's right for you.

Although there are some neat benefits, IF is not for everyone. Your exercise and nutritional experience, and your lifestyle should determine whether you try Intermittent fasting.

Start slowly. Start simply. Start small. Start gradually.

If you decide you'd like to try Intermittent fasting, there's no rush. Pick one small thing to try, even if that's just adjusting regular mealtimes by an hour. Try it. See how it goes.

Focus on what IF approaches have in common, rather than getting bogged down in the details.

Sometimes you eat. Sometimes you don't. That pretty much sums it up.

Know thyself. Observe your own experiences.

Be a scientist. Get started, gather data, gain insight, and draw conclusions that you use to guide future action. Do what's right for you.

Give it time.

There is no rush. Especially since it usually takes a few weeks just to adapt to your new program.

188

Expect ups and downs.

They happen, it's part of life, and it's part of the process. By staying open-minded and not panicking during the "downs," you'll figure out how to have more "ups."

Think about what you genuinely want from Intermittent fasting. Focus on the quality of the process, not the outcome.

Intermittent fasting is a great way to:

- Go deeper into the psychological and physical experience of true hunger;
- Learn the difference between "head hunger" and "body hunger;"
- Learn not to fear hunger;
- Improve insulin sensitivity and re-calibrate your body's use of stored fuel;
- Respect the process and privilege of eating;
- Learn more about your own body;

- Lose fat, if you are careful about it; and,
- Take a break from the work of food prep and the obligation to eat.

IF is not healthy if:

- You're using the pretext of "health" as a way to have an eating disorder or rigidly control your food intake (which is the same thing);
- You fast too often, too long;
- You're also overexercising or not getting enough sleep (i.e., under too much additional physiological stress);
- You're using a lot of supplements, legal or otherwise, to kill your appetite so you can make it through your fasts;
- You're food-obsessed and binge during your non-fasting periods; and,
- You use IF as a way to "compensate" for poor food choices or over-eating.

What you do eat is as important as what you don't.

Get the nutritional basics down first. Eat good quality food, in the right amounts, at the right times. For most people, this is enough to get into great shape. No, Intermittent fasting required.

Respect your body cues.

Pay attention to what your body tells you.

This includes:

- Drastic changes in appetite, hunger, and satiety – including food cravings;
- Sleep quality;
- Energy levels and athletic performance;
- Mood and mental/emotional health;
- Immunity;
- Blood profile;
- Hormonal health; and,
- How you look.

Exercise, but don't overdo it.

We strongly recommend you combine exercise with Intermittent fasting to get the most out of it. Just don't overdo it.

Consider what else is going on in your life.

Think about:

- How much exercise/training you do, and how intensely;
- How well you rest and recover;
- How well IF is fitting into your routine and regular social activities; and,
- What other demands and stress life offer you.

Remember: Intermittent fasting is one of many nutrition styles that work. But it only "works" when it's intermittent, flexible, and part of your routine – not an obligation, and not a constant source of physical and psychological stress.

To help you kick-off your Intermittent Fasting journey in a comfortable, fun, and sustainable (!) way, Here are a 7 Days Intermittent Fasting Plan that gives you action for each day, with a detailed description and more learnings.

Day 1

Today's Task: 12 h Fast | 12 h Eat

Today's Mission: Pick your Intermittent Fasting schedule

During the first week, you want to ease into your Intermittent Fasting slowly. This is why we suggest starting with 12 hours of fasting on your first day, and steady go up to 16 hours on Day 5, by adding 1 additional hour of fasting each day. That way, it is easier for your body and brain to get used to the new way of Eating. Also, you give yourself more time to get used to Intermittent Fasting.

Day 2

Today's Task: 13 h Fast | 11 h Eat

Today's Mission: Learn the basics of Intermittent Fasting

On Day 2, you will be extending your fast to 13 hours. Just one additional hour compared to yesterday – you can do it!

Day 2 is great to get you introduced into healthy eating guidelines that will support your Intermittent Fasting goals: simply focus on eating more whole foods and avoiding the usual suspects such as sugar, processed foods, empty carbs, etc.

Think simple though delicious and balanced meals you can do at home, such as poached eggs with spinach, meatballs with zucchini noodles, feta cheese salad, and homemade hummus for a snack.

Day 3

Today's Task: 14 h Fast | 10 h Eat

Today's Mission: Define your rewards

194

Rewards are crucial when establishing your new Intermittent Fasting habit, hence on Day 3, define your rewards for each successfully fasted day.

Why are rewards so essential?

A reward sends a positive signal to your brain, saying, 'Doing this feels good, we should do more of it!'. It could be anything that makes you feel good.

Ideally, the best Intermittent Fasting reward is related to your primal needs for relaxing, socializing, food, or playing.

Or, your reward could also be a simple (but powerful!) celebratory action you do immediately after completing the habit like cheering yourself up and saying "Good job" or ticking yet another day off of your daily progress tracking sheet you receive when joining the challenge.

If the reward is more significant, for example, dinner at a pricey but so delicious restaurant, you can try token technique – e.g., each successful day fasting 'gives you' 1 token. When you have collected 5 tokens, you get to treat yourself and go out to the restaurant.

Day 4

Today's Task: 15 h Fast | 9 h Eat

Today's Mission: Prepare a high protein lunch

On Day 4 of Intermittent Fasting, you will be fasting for 15 hours already! To break your fast, we recommend having a high protein lunch, which will support your weight loss goals.

For example, you can make yourself steamed or grilled veggies with a protein of your choices, such as grilled meat, poultry, fish, tofu, eggs, beans, legumes or nuts, and seeds.

Day 5

Today's Task: 16 h Fast | 8 h Eat

Today's Mission: Drink black coffee when hungry

On Day 5 of Intermittent Fasting Plan, you will finally be reaching your ultimate 16/8 Intermittent Fasting schedule of fasting for 16 hours and eating within 8 hours window. And it will be pretty easy to achieve, something we have seen ourselves and in hundreds of people that already took the 21 Day Intermittent Fasting challenge.

To help you go through the 16 hours of fasting and curb your hunger, in case you are experiencing one, we recommend drinking black coffee. It is full of antioxidants and is appetite suppressing, too (do not overdo it though!).

Keep in mind: Intermittent Fasting coffee is black coffee. Meaning, don't add any sugar, milk or creamers to it – no cappuccino, latte or flat white, only black coffee.

If you must have something sweet, add natural sweetener stevia, but be careful as it might instigate hunger.

Not a coffee drinker? Go for black or green tea or a glass of water.

Day 6

Today's Task: 16 h Fast | 8 h Eat

Today's Mission: Go for a walk

Are you hoping to lose some pounds during these 7 fasting days? It is essential to stick to a healthy diet, and incorporating some exercise in your routine is recommended.

Go for a walk just before you break your fast. Even a quick 20 min walk will do the trick.

Walking is a great way to improve your overall fitness, your mood, and simply get some fresh air. Most importantly, going for a walk will switch your focus from hunger and help you pass those last hours of fasting easier.

Day 7

Today's Task: 16 h Fast | 8 h Eat

Today's Mission: Go for a walk

Today, keep your new 16/8 Intermittent Fasting Schedule, and while doing so, reflect on your progress from the week.

Reflecting on your progress is part of success – to do so, take a full-body photo, record your weight, and compare them with your starting weight and photo. You should start seeing the first results in your weight and physical appearance.

Also, you can answer a couple of questions to reflect on your progress, such as how do you feel if you have noticed changes in your energy, mood, and skin from Intermittent Fasting, etc.

Going through an exercise like that will help you identify where, and most importantly, why you could be struggling and hence will help you to take action to accelerate your results and make Intermittent Fasting a new sustainable habit.

CHAPTER 13

HOW MUCH WEIGHT CAN YOU LOSE IN A MONTH WITH INTERMITTENT FASTING?

How much will you lose? It depends on how much fasting reduces your average weekly calorie count.

For fun, let's do some an example and see what's possible. We'll call this example Compliant Scarlet.

Example 1 – Complaint Scarlet

Scarlet loves setting goals and hits them every time. Let's see what she can do with 16:8 and a small meal plan.

Let's say right now; she eats about 2100 calories a day on average. She weighs 180 pounds. Friday and Saturday are higher, but she eats a bit less on Sunday, Monday, and Tuesday naturally to balance it out.

She decides to try 16:8. She finds 4-6 meals she likes that she can cook fast.

Each meal is only 500 calories each. Scarlet follows the meal plan below.

- Wakeup – Black coffee or plain tea
- 9 Am Breakfast – 500 calories
- 12 noon Lunch – 500 calories
- 4 PM Dinner – 500 calories
- 5 PM to 9 AM – Fasting

That's 1500 calories for the day.

Scarlet, of course, is compliant all week. So her average calories are 1500 calories a day or 10,500 calories for the week.

"Math Time, Beware! Scarlet is 600 calories under the usual daily intake. 600 over 7 days is 4200 calories. At 3500 calories per pound of fat, that's 4200/3500 or 1.2 pounds of fat loss per week."

She did this for three weeks and felt great. Every Friday morning at precisely 6 AM, she weighed himself before drinking any water and after using the bathroom. Over 3 weeks, she lost 3.6 pounds. She dropped from 180 lbs to 176.4 pounds.

In just 2 more months she's going drop to 166.8. Almost 15 pounds gone. She hasn't seen that on the scale in many years. Plus, she's still dropping.

Example 2 – Jump Around Jill

Now let's look at another scenario. Let's call this one Jumps Around Jill.

Jill's tall and just like Scarlet, she starts at 180 pounds. She, too, wants to drop to 165 pounds before summer. There are a few months to go, and she wants to know if she'll make it.

"Like Scarlet, she eats 2100 calories a day. She knows Scarlet and takes on the same meal plan. She finds 4-6 500 calorie meals that she likes and is easy to make. She even makes them at work."

She follows the same plan:

- Wakeup – Black coffee or plain tea
- 9 Am Breakfast – 500 calories

- 12 noon Lunch – 500 calories
- 4 PM Dinner – 500 calories
- 5 PM to 9 AM – Fasting

Just like Scarlet, she's fast on her way to fat loss.

But then Friday happens... Jill goes out with some friends and has a few drinks. She breaks 16:8 for that night, but it's OK, she says, I've been good all week.

Saturday, she's a bit hungover. One of her friends calls her up and invites her to brunch. She goes. With great intentions, she plans to eat light. But it's chicken and waffles for her. 1500 calories. Just for breakfast. She skips lunch but is ravenous at dinner. Is it hunger or just dehydration from the drinking? It doesn't matter. She drinks a ton of water and gets right back on the meal plan. 500 calorie dinner and starts 16:8 again. She's compliant Sunday too.

Let's see how Jill did. We'll type this up to make it easier to visualize.

Math Time!!!

Monday – 1500 calorie meal plan, 16:8 compliant

Tuesday – 1500 calorie meal plan, 16:8 compliant

Wednesday – 1500 calorie meal plan, 16:8 compliant

Thursday – 1500 calorie meal plan, 16:8 compliant

Friday – 1500 calorie meal plan, 400 calories (4 rum and diet cokes – she was good or was she?), Drinking late means the fasting window was less than 16 hours. 16:8 not compliant.

Saturday – 1500 calorie brunch, 500 calorie dinner. Lots of water.

Sunday – 1500 calorie meal plan, 16:8 compliant

Jill's Totals – 11,400 calories for the week. Before 16:8, she was eating 14,700 calories a week. That's a 3,300 calorie difference. Even with 4 drinks on Friday and Big Brunch Saturday, she still would lose almost a pound that week.

So 16:8 holds up both for Compliant Scarlet and Jumps Around Jill.

Will it work for you? Let's go over 2 more scenarios and find out. Since this section is getting a bit long, I'm going to shorten them.

Both will do 16:8, and both will have a nemesis. Can they defeat their nemesis? Let's find out.

Example 3 – Christmas Joy

Christmas Joy is on track most of the year. She follows 16:8 and is at her goal weight of 165 pounds.

Christmas is her favorite and also his overeating nemesis.

She never has and never will hold back through the holidays.

She knows this. She makes a plan. You can probably see how this will turn out!

Like Jill and Scarlet, Joy has a 1500 calorie a day meal plan and follows 16:8. That's 10,500 calories a week, and it keeps her at 165 lbs.

Christmas rolls around, and Joy has a massive 6,000 calorie meal that night. She also ate her usual breakfast and lunch. She's a man of habit! Her total for the day is 7000 calories!

It looks like Joy didn't make it, or did she? Sounds like its...

Math Time!!!

Joy's weekly total is 16,000 calories. How much weight did she gain? 16,000 for the week minus 10500 average for the week divided by 3500 calories per pound gives us an extra 5500 calories for the week. That's a gain of 1.6 pounds gained for the week.

Is all hope lost? No, Carl planned for this. She's been doing 16:8 for months. She's practiced fasting, and she's good at it. She's also done some 24 and 36-hour fasts now and then. She knows to stay busy and other methods to help him get through a longer fast.

The week before Thanksgiving, she did a 36 hour fast on Monday (eat Sunday, skip Monday, normal Tuesday – 36 hours from Sunday dinner to Tuesday breakfast). She did another one that last Thursday. That's 1500 calories over two days she didn't eat, or 3000 calories total. That's not enough to make up the 5500.

Again, Joy planned for this. She also plans to do the same on Monday and Thursday the week after Thanksgiving. She knows 36 hour fasts are hard, but so is giving up this 165 lb body she loves!

Plus, she knows she only has to do those longer fasts 4 times.

So she does them. She's down 6000 calories. Problem solved. Joy stayed at 165 pounds all season using a combination of 16:8 and targeted 36-hour fasts.

Nothing lost, but nothing gained. Joy makes it through the holiday season with no net weight gain with some carefully timed fasts.

Three success stories so far, but we have one more contestant to go. Meet Party Pete.

Example 4 – Party Mary

Party Mary loves to Party. For Mary, every week is Thanksgiving.

There's a holiday going on somewhere!

Mary's best friend is Joy. May watches maintain 165 lbs every holiday season, no matter how much Joy eats.

May wants to do the same. Her nemesis, Mary, loves to party all the time.

Like Joy, Mary's started 16:8 and is on a roll. Like Joy, Mary worked his way up to 36-hour fasts. She learned what she had to do to stay compliant and distracted to get through the longer fasts.

Unlike Joy, Mary still has a least 1-2 party nights a week. Either she drinks too much or overeats.

So does Mary make it? Let's see. It sounds like it's...

Math Time!!!

Monday – 1500 calorie meal plan, 16:8 compliant

Tuesday – 1500 calorie meal plan, 16:8 compliant

Wednesday – 1500 calorie meal plan, 600 calories – Happy hour, light beer only, fasting 12 hours

Thursday – 1500 calorie meal plan, 16:8 compliant

Friday – 1500 calorie meal plan, 1500 calorie burger and fries, 1000 calories Friday night out (mixed of different drinks), Fasting only from 1:30 Am to 9 Am on Saturday

Saturday – Massive hangover. 1500 calorie dinner breakfast followed by hangry 500 calorie lunch and 500 calorie dinner. 16:8 complaint

Sunday – 1500 calorie meal plan, 16:8 compliant

Mary's totals – 14,600 calories for the week (16:8 fasting only). Like the others, Mary's previous daily was 2100 calories a day or 14700. She's under but not enough. Due to errors in estimating how much she eats, Mary's weight stays at 180 for 2 months.

Mary hates 16:8. He talks to Joy. Joy talks about the 36-hour fasts. Mary gives it a try.

Let's see if longer fasts help, even with all that partying.

Monday – 36 hour fast (0), 16:8 compliant

Tuesday – 1500 calorie meal plan, 16:8 compliant

Wednesday – 1500 calorie meal plan, 600 calories – Happy hour, light beer only, fasting 12 hours

Thursday – 36 hour fast (0), 16:8 compliant

Friday – 1500 calorie meal plan, 1500 calorie burger and fries, 1000 calories Friday night out (mixed of different drinks), Fasting only from 1:30 Am to 9 Am on Saturday

Saturday – Massive hangover. 1500 calorie dinner breakfast followed by hangry 500 calorie lunch and 500 calorie dinner. 16:8 complaint

Sunday – 1500 calorie meal plan, 16:8 compliant

Mary's totals – 11,600 calories for the week (with 36-hour fasts). Like the others, Mary's previous daily was 2100 over 7 days or 14,700 calories a week. Mary finally starts losing weight! She's down 3100 calories or almost a pound.

Mary feels freaking, invincible. 1 pound a week. This is Party Mary here! She does nothing halfhearted.

She's going to set this fat on fire!

Now she starts 36-hour fasts two days after every binge. Let's see how it panned out over 2 weeks.

Week 1

Monday – 36 hour fast (0)

Tuesday – 2100 calories – Normal meal plan plus small binge. Just a quick happy hour with friends.

Wednesday – 36 hour fast (0) – Thursday's coming, and it's the new Friday!

Thursday – 1500 calorie meal plan, 1500 calorie dinner, 1000 calories drinks. I'm invincible with fasting!

Friday – Hangover. 1000 calories – Eats 2 meal plan meals for breakfast. 500 calorie lunch and 500 calorie Dinner. But...1500 calorie happy hour and 750 calories for 3 slices of late-night pizza.

Saturday – Massive hangover. 1500 calorie dinner breakfast followed by hangry 500 calorie lunch and 500 calorie dinner.

Sunday – 36 hour fast (0)

Totals for Week 1 – 12,850. 14,700 – 12850 / 3500 = Pete lost ½ a pound. Success still!

Week 2

Monday – 1500 calorie meal plan, 16:8 compliant

Tuesday – 36 hr fast (0)

Wednesday – 1500 calorie meal plan, 1500 calorie binge

Thursday – 36 hr fast (0)

Friday – 1500 calorie meal plan, 1500 calorie binge

Saturday – 1500 calorie brunch, 500 calorie lunch, 500 calorie dinner, 1500 calorie binge

Sunday – 36 hr fast (0) – extremely difficult. Lots of sicknesses

Totals for Week 2 – 11,500. 14700 – 11500 / 3500 = Pete loses another pound. Success again!

But is this a success? Can you see the pattern here? How long do you think Pete can hold out?

She may be losing weight, but he may be heading for an eating disorder. Binge and purge. Binge and purge.

Mary's heading towards bulimia. This is a serious condition. Whether you purge from vomiting, laxatives, or fasting, it's all the same.

If you're bouncing back and forth from big eats to no eats, you may have a problem. This is the dark side of fasting. Fasting is powerful. Yes, you can lose a ton of weight. Yes, you can eat what you like. But if you're not careful, it will own you. Just like junk food addiction, you can have a fasting addiction.

If you or someone you know is going down this path, please seek help. It's serious. People die from eating disorders.

Fasting. Keto. Paleo. Calorie Counting. These are powerful tools. Depending on the person, they can work great. They can also be a huge detriment to your life.

Respect your body and the tools you use to change it. You can have the body of your dreams. You deserve it.

You don't need to set that fat on fire to get the results you want. Just go slowly, pay attention, and get feedback from friends you trust that have gone there before you.

Does Your Body Burn Fat Or Muscle First When Fasting?

Both mostly fat. Many studies have been done on this. On the first day of a fast, there is a small, small amount of muscle burn along with the fat.

Then your body will dump human growth hormone, which stops the burning of muscle. It does that to conserve muscle.

Think about it. We have gone through fasting periods naturally as part of our evolution. There wasn't always a 7-11 nearby. If the body were designed to burn muscle during a fast, we wouldn't have the energy to go out and find more food.

The result of that – extinction.

So instead, we use fat as our long term energy storage and emergency energy supply.

This is why fasting is so great. It's the best way to tap into our fat stores and burn them away. Combined with a compliant meal plan and you're ready to light that fat on a fire.

CHAPTER 14
INTERMITTENT FASTING VERSUS OTHER DIETS

Any diet that makes someone go without food for some time is known as I intermittent fasting. When you compare intermittent fasting with the 3-day diet, which is also known as the military diet due to its strictness, you will see their differences. Unlike intermittent fasting, where you can eat after a few hours, in the 3-day diet you go for three days fasting, and the remaining four days you can go back to healthy eating. It is also a very low-fat diet that helps people shed weight extremely fast due to the lack of calories. Unlike intermittent fasting, with the 3-day fasting, calories will come back full force when the calorie period is over. It also does not provide the nutrients needed by the body because of the intake of the required amount of fruits and vegetables is strictly limited, unlike in intermittent fasting.

A master cleanse lemonade diet is also another diet plan that helps in weight loss. Unlike the intermittent where you can have meals at stipulated times, the master cleanses lemonade diet only allows you to drink a beverage that resembles lemonade and salt water through the ten days. Intermittent fasting has significant health benefits, but the same cannot be said for the masters cleanse lemonade diet. This is because, during the ten days, you will not take the required amount of calories or nutrients that boost the immunity of the body, and the calorie intake is restricted to 650 only. Unlike in the intermittent fasting diet where your cravings and eating habits may be improved, in the master cleanse diet, you may end up overeating after the diet plan and gain even more weight.

Fast diet is different from intermittent fasting in that a person is not allowed to have a heavy meal during the eating window. That is why some people find it hard to follow religiously. With the fast day diet, it is almost impossible to get your daily required nutrients. That is because even calorie intake is supposed to be less than 500 in women and less than 600 in men that will only meet your daily energy limit. The good thing about intermittent fasting is that during the eating window, you do not have to count the calories you consume, making it a preferable diet. Studies carried out suggested that unlike the fast meal plan, intermittent fasting increased longevity in both men and women and had more health benefits.

Intermittent fasting shopping list

For the first three days of fasting, you will need to shop for the following food items.

i. Fish

It is essential to include fish in your shopping list. This is because it usually contains healthy fats and proteins the right amount of vitamin D. Your meals should be packed with more nutrients. They will help your body and fish will ensure you get them, including feeding your brain.

ii. Potatoes

Potatoes are one of the best foods in making someone full. This is because it takes minimum effort for the body to digest. During intermittent fasting, vegetables are essential, especially when cooled it forms a starch primed resistance which helps in fueling good bacteria found in the gut.

iii. Berries.

Vitamin C, which is used in the boosting of the immune system, is found in strawberries. Studies suggest that when added to your intermittent fasting diet, it can help in the reduction of your body mass index over 14 years. This is thanks to vital nutrients such as flavonoids.

iv. Nuts

Nuts have been known to remove body fat and help in longevity and reduce the risk of cardiovascular illnesses such as type 2 diabetes. The presence of polyunsaturated fats in nuts can help a person to feel fuller for long hours.

v. Eggs.

Eggs usually contain proteins which are essential during intermittent fasting as it will keep the body full for longer hours and help in the building of muscles. A study that was carried out showed that when some men ate a bagel for breakfast, they tended to be more hungry than their counterparts that fed on eggs for breakfast. This made them feed on more calories throughout the day, causing them to lose very minimal weight.

vi. Whole grains.

Whole grains are one of the items that should be included in your shopping list when doing intermittent fasting. This is because they contain vibrant levels of protein and fiber, making a person feel full for long hours. Whole grains like lentils are perfect when it comes to iron, which is very important, especially for women who are fasting.

vii. Salmon

Salmon is another critical item to include on your intermittent fasting shopping list because of its links with longevity. Salmon also has high levels of EPA and DHA, which are the omega-three fatty acids that boost the brain functions.

viii. Fortified vitamin D milk

Fortified vitamin D milk is vital because it highly increases the capability of the body to absorb calcium. The calcium helps the bones, and the good thing is that you can use it in your cereals or even smoothies.

ix. Pawpaw

Pawpaw is one of the critical items that you have to include in your shopping list. This is because it contains essential enzymes known as papain that are usually used to break down proteins. These enzymes help reducing issues caused by overeating such as bloating, especially when you just started intermittent fasting and you go for hours without eating.

x.   Water.

Water is one of the essential items on the list because it helps you stay hydrated for the excellent health and optimum function of almost all organs in the body. Dehydration causes fatigue and lightheadedness. You will expel dark yellow urine, which is very smelly, and when you can go through this with unlimited food, it can be hazardous.

Intermittent fasting can be used as a weight-loss tool, and above all, it has very many health benefits. Below is an intermittent fasting meal plan that will see to it that you have a smooth fast.

i. 9 am- black tea

When doing the intermittent fasting, most of your eating habits will change, and this is because you will have to accommodate healthier meals and beverages. Taking black tea is healthy because it is a calorie-free drink.

ii. 11 am -1.30pm mild workout and lots of water.

At this time, you are required to drink lots of water and stay busy. When you remain idle, it is very easy, falling into temptation and binge eating is very easy. Try and be as active as you can be. Mild exercises such as walking, doing house chores that keep you busy until your eating window. Being proactive will help your mind to be more alert.

iii. 2pm–3.30 pm drink sparkling water

When you are almost finishing your fast, and you have a strong urge to have something more than water in your tummy. You can go for sparkling water. It usually has zero calories and makes one feel fuller for longer. This is advantageous because when you feel full, you will not crave for unhealthy meals.

iv. 4 pm breaking of the fast.

You can use a low-calorie protein bar and a fruit to break your fast. Apples are the most preferred fruit for breaking a fast as they low in calorie, and the larger capacity is water. Apples are also very palatable and make someone stay fuller for longer, and the good news is it contains minimal calories. Apple also have carbohydrates that

v. 4.30 pm – 7 pm

When you snack in the afternoon, your body may start to feel hungrier. The calorie intake for the afternoon snack should be less than 500 calories. All you need to do is be patient to let the food you ate before to start providing energy for the body. You do not have to take more snacks, be active, and try not to think about the hunger so much. Try and run some errands or work on some projects as you wait for the energy to start being produced.

vi. 7.30pm meal time.

At this time, you can now pay yourself off by having one hearty meal. You are allowed to have a substantial amount of food. The meal is supposed to be your primary calorie source, so this means that you have to eat a well-balanced meal. You are not only supposed to have a big meal but to also make sure there is a right balance of macronutrients. The level of proteins should be higher than fat and carbohydrates, which should be taken in moderation. Every meal should at least contain less than 1000 calories. Some of the foods you can take during a meal are rice, white meat either fish of skinned chicken, vegetables, and some cheese which will provide fat content in the feed. Another simple, quick meal that you can consume during your eating period is pasta, minced meat with some vegetables of your choice. When you decide to go out for dinner, you can always order food that has the same nutrients as the ones discussed above but still try and eat moderately.

vii. At 11 pm you can have your dessert.

After your meal, you can have one last dessert before going to bed. Your last snack should be high in protein, but less than 400 calories, and this is dependent on the number of calories you have had during the day.

This works like magic every time you fast. It is ok to try your recipes as long as they are healthy. If they contain all the required nutrients, you are good to go. You should at least try and not go above 2000 calories per day because it might be too much.

Some people might choose to bulk when doing intermittent fasting. Bulking has benefits such as increased human growth hormones that help with the growth of muscles. It can also increase insulin sensitivity, which will, in turn, make your gains leaner. Recent studies concluded that when you lose weight, you can easily preserve your muscle mass. When bulking, your body will need more calories than the one found in the meal plan shown above, so in that case, all you need to do is add more calories. Foods that will help with this are oatmeal, Greek yogurt, and at times, cheese quesadilla.

The Most Frequently Questioned Products

The below list provides you answers to the most frequently questioned products and summarizes the effects they have on intermittent fasting.

Products are listed in the order from the most preferred to the least preferred during your fasting period.

E.g., Mineral water is the most preferred option for Intermittent Fasting drinks, while Almond milk is the least favorite.

Mineral Water

Mineral water and water, in general, are free of calories and allowed during fasting. Mineral water is full of minerals to help restore electrolyte and mineral imbalance that happens while fasting. For this reason, mineral water is the most advisable Intermittent Fasting drink.

Coffee

Coffee is allowed during fasting hours, and in fact, some studies have shown that it may support the fat burning and reduce insulin sensitivity over time. For many people, it also acts as an appetite suppressant, hence it is an excellent choice for those fasted hungry mornings.

Too much caffeine, however, can harm your body, hence do not overdo the recommended daily dose of 400 mg of caffeine (2-2.5 cups of brewed coffee) for healthy adults.

Apple Cider Vinegar

Does apple cider vinegar break a fast?

Apple cider vinegar is free of calories and allowed during fasting. It helps to lower blood sugar levels and improve digestion when following Intermittent Fasting.

How to use it? Drink 1-2 tbsp of apple cider vinegar diluted in water. Particularly, drinking it before a meal can aid digestion and increase the feeling of fullness.

Stevia

Stevia is a natural sweetener and a right choice if you must have something sweet. Studies have shown that it has no adverse side effects as compared to artificial sweeteners and might even lover glucose and insulin levels. It might, however, instigate hunger for some, and you might want to be careful.

Coconut Oil

Coconut oil and other oils contain pure fats. Technically speaking, anything that has calories, even if it is a tiny amount, break your fast. However, fat has little to no effect on insulin, blood glucose, or any of the other measurements that indicate a "broken fast." For this reason, it could be considered as part of fasting, as popularized by Bulletproof fasting.

If you prefer 'clean' fasting though, you should try to sustain from consuming any oils and butter, and hence sustain from Bulletproof coffee during your fasting hours. Also, note that fats are incredibly high in calories; therefore, you should keep this in mind if you are trying to lose weight.

Butter

Butter is pure fat, the same as coconut oil. It also has little to no effect on insulin and could be allowed while fasting (e.g., by drinking bulletproof coffee). However, the same as coconut oil, it is extremely high in calories.

Almond Milk

Does Almond milk break a fast? Technically speaking, YES! However, if you absolutely must have something and are OK with 'open fasting (read more in our 'Cheat Sheet you can download below) - a splash of almond milk can be a good alternative.

Almond milk is low in carbs and calories, hence up to 0.5 cup/100 ml of almond milk could be a good vegan option for 'open fasting.' When choosing almond milk, avoid the ones with added sugar or those fortified with extra protein.

Bone Broth

Bone Broth usually is very low in calories and carbs but does contain protein, which technically breaks the fast, fat burning and autophagy. Some experts do, however, allow bone broth on exceptional cases (up to 20 kcal per fasting period), especially since it helps to replenish the salt lost while not eating.

Artificial Sweeteners

There is a lot of conflicting information and different studies done around artificial sweeteners and their effects on the health and insulin response. While some studies show that artificial sweeteners such as aspartame, saccharin, or sucralose do not raise insulin, they might disrupt the balance of gut bacteria in some people.

Given the uncertainty and ongoing debates on the effects of artificial sweeteners. The most common brand names of artificial sweeteners are Splenda (sucralose), Nutrasweet, Equal or Sugar Twin (aspartame), Sweet'N Low (saccharin).

Frequently Asked Questions

i. How will intermittent fasting slow down aging?

Intermittent fasting has been proved to help people from the risks of cardiovascular diseases. These and other conditions or risk factors that are age-related like Alzheimer's disease by lowering the inflation in the brain protecting the nerve cells is also a benefit of intermittent fasting. Studies that were carried out on animals showed that intermittent fasting activated autophagy that is the process of the cells in the body breaks down dysfunctional cells. It helps in the secretion of the human growth hormones that boost the process of burning fat.

ii. Is it ok to exercise while fasting?

For beginners, it is advisable to exercise less because the body does not have enough energy. A study showed that those who did exercise while fasting lost more weight than those who did not. When your fasting window is at night, then a morning exercise before breakfast is advisable. This is because then, your body will burn more fat due to the depletion of glycogen.

iii. Is intermittent fasting safe?

Many people have benefited from practicing intermittent fasting, especially the shorter ones which are less than 24 hours. This, however, does not mean that it is safe for everyone. Pregnant women, children, and people who have type 1 diabetes are not advised to fast.

iv. What is intermittent fasting?

Intermittent fasting is the use of cycles to fast and eat to lose weight and for other health benefits such as cardiovascular health. Studies have shown that intermittent fasting can help in the reduction of chronic illnesses such as diabetes type 2. Other diseases are hypertension and even diseases that affect the brain negatively, such as Alzheimer's disease.

v. Is it ok to take supplements during fasting?

Taking supplements when fasting is ok when fasting.

vi. How many types of intermittent fasting do we have?

There are many different types of intermittent fasting, but the most common ones are the 12-hour fasting and 12-hour eating window. This is the most advised fasting method for beginners. The 16/8 way is another method that involves fasting for 16 hours in a day and restricting your eating for the remaining 8 hours. There is also the 5:2 diet. It is the method whereby you limit your calorie intake to 600 maximum on two days of the week, which does not have to be consecutive. Then the other standard way is the 24-hour fasting whereby you go for a whole day without eating. For example, when you eat supper today, you wait up to the next day from you to eat.

vii. Can intermittent fasting help a diabetic person?

Research has shown that intermittent fasting can help in the reduction of suffering from diabetes type 2. That is because fasting will lower blood sugar levels and reduce insulin resistance.

viii. Does fasting affect your hormones?

Intermittent fasting can positively affect your hormones because during a fast, the level of hormones such as the human growth hormones improved by almost five times. It also causes the cells to repair themselves, thus removing the old ones that are not functioning well and replacing them with ones that work correctly.

CONCLUSION

Intermittent fasting is a tool that can be very useful when it comes to weight loss and other health benefits. Unlike other weight-loss diets that are extremely hard to follow, which all failed you in the past, intermittent fasting will give you a reliable option that will positively affect your life. The most popular advantage of intermittent fasting that makes it the best weight-loss tool is that you can enjoy your bottle of wine. All the freshly baked cakes, and cookies and you will not have to turn your friends and family down when they invite you to events because of the fear of backsliding from your journey because you can have all you want during your eating window just that you indulge moderately. The good thing about Intermittent fasting is that it is a very straight forward and easy to follow a diet that will change your life for the better. All the useful techniques and mistakes to avoid when fasting can help with going through the diet without any hitches. As we have seen, intermittent fasting is extremely beneficial for the body, especially health-wise. Healthy individuals should do intermittent fasting at least once to get all the benefits that come with intermittent fasting. You can easily make intermittent fasting part of your day to day life. If you find that you keep failing, all you need to do is reduce your fasting window and keep going.

FOR MY MOTHER

Mely Johnson

Made in the USA
Coppell, TX
26 April 2020

22396312R00134